Biosecurity in the Making
The Threats, the Aspects and the Challenge of Readiness

Editor

Manousos E. Kambouris
University of Patras, School of Health Sciences
Department of Pharmacy, Patras, Greece

and

The Golden Helix Foundation
London, United Kingdom

CRC Press
Taylor & Francis Group
Boca Raton London New York

CRC Press is an imprint of the
Taylor & Francis Group, an **informa** business

A SCIENCE PUBLISHERS BOOK

Cover credit

- The hand microscope and the fungus image, are from the collection of Ret Prof. Velegraki, one of the authors (Chapters 2, 5).
- The UAV over the agricultural exploitation image, is from the collection of Dr. Manoussopoulos, co-author in Chapters 2, 6.
- The electromicrobiology setup image, is from the collection of LaPIT/Dept of Pharmacy/ University of Patras, headed by Prof. Patrinos, also co-author of Chapter 5.

First edition published 2024
by CRC Press
2385 NW Executive Center Drive, Suite 320, Boca Raton FL 33431

and by CRC Press
4 Park Square, Milton Park, Abingdon, Oxon, OX14 4RN

CRC Press is an imprint of Taylor & Francis Group, LLC

Library of Congress Cataloging-in-Publication Data (applied for)

ISBN: 978-1-032-27732-5 (hbk)
ISBN: 978-1-032-27733-2 (pbk)
ISBN: 978-1-003-29384-2 (ebk)

DOI: 10.1201/9781003293842

Typeset in Times New Roman
by Radiant Productions

Preface

The issue of Bio-hostilities (Biowarfare, Bioterrorism and Biocrime) seems to accompany tacitly the human history since always; but it emerges to prominence, even if hidden or masqueraded, in certain sociopolitical conditions. These are not readily identifiable, but one may bet that this generation of humans does witness one. It is the subtlety of the tool at a time of massively effective weapons in an interconnected planetary civilization. It is the progress afforded by proprietary research into corporate labs and affiliated institutions. It is the enabling by other technologies, such as Informatics. Or it is all of the above, and many others. The threat is real, and this book was conceived before the COVID-19. The pandemic made the book all the more relevant in current times and proved the basic issue: that biosecurity must be taken seriously. The hows and whys of this new struggle for freedom have primed this book, which seems to have arrived a tad late for serving as a warning; however, it is handy for assimilation of lessons and management of liabilities for future reference.

Dedicated to the teachings and memory of Professor E. M. Kambouris, who, in the late 80s, fortuitously spoke the nature of Things to Come.

Contents

Preface		iii
Introduction		vii

1. **A (hi)story of Horror: Biosociomics as an Integrated Field**   **1**
   to Critically Research the Occurrence of Biothreats throughout the Ages
   M.E. Kambouris, Y. Manoussopoulos, A. Velegraki and G.P. Patrinos

2. **Agrosecurity: Integrating the Containment of Agroterrorism,**   **16**
   Promotion of Bioeconomy and Protection of the Public Health
   Yiannis Manoussopoulos, Aristea Velegraki, Marianna Manoussopoulou
   and *Manousos E. Kambouris*

3. **The Enemy in the Dish: Current and Projected Foodborne**   **29**
   Biorisks and Liabilities
   M. Kakagianni and I. Giavasis

4. **Beyond the Biosphere**   **49**
   M.E. Kambouris

5. **Nature Avenging**   **66**
   Manousos E. Kambouris, Aristea Velegraki and George P. Patrinos

6. **The Enemy Within: Turning the Pages**   **93**
   M.E. Kambouris and Y. Manoussopoulos

7. **The Hope of Biologicals: Toxins, Microbiomes and Phages**   **107**
   M.E. Kambouris

8. **Cyberbiosecurity: The Threat of the Sages**   **119**
   Ioannis Chatzis, Periklis Rompolas, Christoforos Karachristos and
   Angeliki Grivopoulou

9. **Harnessing Fields, Waves and Currents: The Realm of Mages**   **133**
   M.E. Kambouris

10. **Wars, Crime and Terror: The Perpetrated Dimension of Biothreats**   **150**
    George D. Kostis and Manousos E. Kambouris

Index   **167**

Introduction

What is that thing?

Biosecurity as an official concept has been promoted for less than two decades. It was a legitimate concept used by experts and became widely known as a means for providing a politically correct mantle for anything reminding of biological warfare and bioterrorism, in the wake of the bioterrorism events at the dawn of the 21st century, especially the Anthrax letters in the US and the alleged weapons of mass destruction (especially bioweapons) of Baathist Iraq in 2003. The public had been sensitized on such threats by the revelation of the gigantic Project Vector of the later decades of the USSR. This became publically known to the rest of the World thanks to defecting insiders. Additional sensitization of the public was caused by the realization that in the last decade of the 20th century, bioterrorism and biowarfare incidents had taken place, away from the lights of publicity: the former case is exemplified by the unsuccessful attacks of the Aum Shinrikyo in Japan, before the Sarin incident; the latter is exemplified by the alleged use of mycotoxins in 1991, against coalition troops, by the Iraqis, as a revenge measure. Many other cases, from biocrimes (use of bioagents for targeted assassinations by state and non-state agents) to proper bio- and agroterrorism are less well-substantiated.

Biowarfare, as a framework of activities, was banned by a series of international conventions; however, they failed singularly in preventing a number of countries of special international status from engaging in such activities; the countries referred to included both highly esteemed ones as well as those bereft of any esteem altogether— practically of pariah status (possibly Libya and North Korea). This created a just as legitimate need to promote research and acquisition initiatives towards known and, which is the key, projected threats. The way to prioritize the projected portion of the threats meant a tacit approval for experimentation on offensive agents for defensive purposes, allegedly to assess their potential and pinpoint the liabilities of possible use, thus creating blueprints for countermeasures in both material and procedural levels. Among such approaches, the 'gain-of-function', as recently termed, is a proper, in all but name, development of offensive biowarfare agents with only the scale of production and the intended use setting it apart from bioweapons' development.

Both these issues are debatable: biowarfare needs some minimum mass, but bioterrorism not so much. Additionally, the proliferating agents cast a shadow of doubt on the concept of 'mass production' as complex mathematics *may* define massiveness in terms of results and not of the mass/quantity of the released agent.

Many cases of biosecurity response start with 'patient 0', and while 'Patient 1' may be a better idea, the whole concept remains valid: it all starts with one host and, possibly, with one altered particle of the agent, or of the productive unit of the said agent, if the agent is not alive or, actually, not propagating.

Although the term *Biosecurity* is relatively new, the concept is indeed old and has proven to be important through the course of ages. Disease or, rather, plague (*sensu lato*) has been a major factor in shaping both environmental and human populations. Its importance in changing the route of history is clearly substantiated through the American history, where massive depopulation of the natives assisted the *Conquistadors*, through the recasting of the political system in Europe after the Black Death and the fall of the Athenian empire. Pestilence is one of the Knights of the Apocalypse precisely because it has the potential to bring about existential-scale events, currently included in the GCBR (Global Catastrophic Biological Risks) category. Although a mere pestilence may be local in planetary terms and thus not qualify as a GCBR, the disruptive effect may amplify the catastrophic potential to GCBR proportions and impact in a very networked planet.

Famine is another factor just as destructive and just as historical; the depopulation of Ireland due to famine is attributable to an agrosecurity lapse that resulted in the failure of the potato crop, amplified by ecological and aggravated by sociopolitical factors. In Germany on the other hand, the introduction of potato, being more robust than wheat, assisted in resolving the problem of sufficiency in basic foodstuff/food security and fueled the explosive growth of the industry and an increase in population. Thus, anything curtailing the possibility of a famine outbreak is a matter of biosecurity of the highest priority. With this background, it is evident that failures in foodstuff production, an issue of biosecurity by definition, may also have *direct* biological causes, including infectious diseases of different kinds—along with the natural enemies of the used productive organisms. The effects of food shortages caused by non-agrosecurity reasons in the last 3 decades bear witness to the magnitude of the danger and of the degree of vulnerability: the first food crisis was entirely a result of misuse of resources due to the use of plants intended for biofuels instead of edible produce - especially low-cost and thus widely needed produce such as soy, rice, corn and wheat. The ultimate crisis was to result from the massive use of land for direct production of energy by planting solar panels, once more at the expense of food-producing exploitations, while the leveraging of the market by the diminished foodstuff export in 2022, due to the events in Ukraine, manifested a magnified supply chain crisis originally due to the COVID-19 disruption.

Public Health had been correctly identified as a matter of state security early on, and not only in terms of welfare (the Greeks had established state-sponsored health provisions at least since early 5th century); the biosector in general was used actively to enact political effects: The Greek mythology directly states the impact of animal and human epidemics and plant diseases on the security of the realm and of the royal houses. The Old Testament corroborates this, especially with the seven years of famine in Egypt. Still, the concept of biosecurity extending to practically engulf all lifeforms and habitats on the planet, and treated prospectively as a cause of War—for all practical purposes - is indeed innovative. Trying to cause zoonoses to undermine an enemy's ability to wage war had been officially endorsed by the

Germans in World War I; to starve the enemy into surrender had been a British plan against the Germans in WW II, and an American one against the Koreans in the 1950s; it was also the reason behind the slaughter of the buffaloes in the 19th century, with the support of and subsidy from the US Army, so as to exhaust the major food resource of 'unruly' and independent-minded native tribes. The interdependence of political status, especially in terms of regime stability or social unrest and the welfare and health of its living, growing resources, for any kind and number of applications, is well established today as it was since ancient times.

A direct conceptual outcrop of the Digital Planet and of Globalization, the concept of biosecurity, *as projected today*, has a strong component of perpetrated human agency, perhaps unduly so. This is because it blossomed in the cinders of massive terror attacks. The latter were conventional (as in the Twin Towers and the Madrid Rail Attacks) as well as unconventional (as in the Tokyo subway or the Anthrax Letters in the US). As a result, from the bioterrorism/counterbioterrorism (Chapter 10) and agroterrorism (Chapter 2) concepts of the 1990s and 2000s to the idea of biocrime and the inclusive notion of biosecurity today, the idea of an expanded awareness and intervention scheme to guard against threats stemming from biological entities has reached a rather mature context. Today, it further evolves to keep up with the possible novel threats and risk factors. The maturity reflects, most of all, the understanding of multi-dimensional connectivity, with health issues considered as the digits of a mosaic encompassing the planet, or rather the biosphere and practically all the communities of the Living.

Biothreats were integrated into the hybrid (or the regular) warfare agenda in the two World Wars, a fact not widely known. Contrary to the spectacular and devastating use of chemicals in the First and the conspicuous absence of chemical agents during the Second, biowarfare was discreet but, in some cases, decisive and fully embedded in the operational doctrines. The massive infection by injection of cavalry mounts and equine transport haulers by the Imperial German agents cannot be understood but within the greater context of WW I, where cavalry was the maneuver arm expected to exploit any breakthrough in the trench warfare, and the transportation of ammunition and supplies was focal in achieving such a decisive result or denying it to the enemy. The use of Typhus in WW II, in Stalingrad, by the Soviets, was assisted by frightful conditions—especially the dearth of supplies, including medical supplies of course—and targeted at degrading the fighting edge of an enemy clearly superior, at least in tactics, morale, experience and training.

One must take a moment to ponder upon the Plague of Athens, the reason for the fall of the Athenian empire; despite the plague, it took some luck and more than two decades to topple the plague-stricken state. It would be logical to suppose that without the plague, the empire would have emerged victorious. Its opponents, especially those unseen, might have drawn similar conclusions and thus followed the—ancient—example of the—Athenian—Solon; it is possible, if not outright probable, that they *did* used Biology as a weapon. They may have, or not; but the Athenians definitely thought so.

The temptation to destroy the food resources, as a weapon of mass destruction, was not lost to modern and ancient leaders. There are many cases of prominent droughts in ancient literature, that were miraculously resolved when a condition—

usually a divine prerogative—was met or satisfied; droughts were not necessarily associated with weather and raining. A developed concept suggests considering, as options, first the agrowarfare, perhaps initiated by British plans to destroy the German agricultural base in WW II so as to multiply the effect of the naval blockade; and then a concerted effort against wildlife as well. If nothing else, oxygen supply is diminished by wildfires and desertification progresses due to the loss of soil by rainfalls. It is a long-term but valid plan, rarely taken into consideration but actively pursued, in the mainland and archipelagic Greece during the tensions with some of its neighbors since the 1970s: for instance, Turkish agents have been recorded to acknowledge this fact, and some arrests of other nationals showed the extent of planning of such operations, despite the very real internal dimension of land appropriation for urban expansion and livestock breeding.

Although the issue of endangered species and biodiversity has been something of a taboo for much of the world in the past decades, it must be understood that Nature does not see it that way. The number of species that would be extinct before humanity starts taking a toll on the biodiversity is incalculable; dinosaurs are but one example. Biodiversity is no means by itself; it was intended for a purpose, elusive to human intelligence. Once this purpose was obsolete, biodiversity would have no place in the blueprint of evolution. Quite possibly, (part of) this purpose was to guard against randomness by increasing adaptability in a collective context. If no evolutionary pressure is on, biodiversity has no existential reason. And this is the most probable causative agent behind the threat of existential level events. There is no reason for this not to happen. A species may be vital for the survival of another; thus, if one goes, so might the other. This is inconsequential. A whole network may be deleted actually; however, other species will step up and new ones may emerge. The extinction of the dinosaurs gave ecological room to the mammals. The whales would have been extinct if the Megalodons had not, in the first place. In some cases, there is not enough room for two, and this is not simply a matter of uniqueness of the ecological niche. It is much more interactive; many species have hunted their prey to extinction, to follow suit or to simply find another. Thus, there is no natural tendency for conservation of species, and extinction level events are not difficult to happen, for they are not thermodynamically unfavorable or discouraged by any sort of providence, safety mechanism or counterbalancing routine.

How did you say it works?

The implementation of biosecurity requires a cognitive process based on a number of questions—some rather simple, and others of growing complexity; the answers to these questions interdepend in various ways, based on not only the questions themselves, but also the spatio-temporal and actual continuum; different degrees of interdependence may be expected in different occurrences.

The first such question is a rather predictable one: What/Which? It clearly refers to the nature and identity (in this order) of the deleterious/detrimental/infectious agent, a piece of information affecting the impact, the disease dynamics in terms of dissemination, the diagnostics and the response (therapy/disinfection). Obviously, live agents are much more important to identify in order to predict dissemination and transmittance, compared to molecular or biochemical agents (such as toxins). It is important to highlight that the biochemical agents originally included (bio)toxins and bioregulators (the toxin being a specific case of bioregulators actually), but the possibility of eDNA (for "environmental DNA") and other classes of agents affecting the genomic content and the genetic processes and dynamics makes the rather wider category, 'biomolecular', handier for such inclusive considerations.

To answer the What/Which query is not simply a matter of identification of an agent through a process of taxonomy as usually understood in medical microbiology. It might be much more basic- and also complicated; for example, is the cause of a syndrome/disease a molecular agent, such as toxin, eDNA or bioregulator? Or is it a microbial one—and then what kind of the latter? Parasite, fungus, bacterium, or virus? Might it be a prion perhaps?

The process of identification may be informed when presupposing the identity of an agent (or, occasionally, one from a panel of several possibilities) and confirming or rejecting the presupposition by means of the analytical evidence—usually results of some diagnostic test, as in the testing process for SARS-CoV-2. Or it may be agnostic—for instance when there is no presupposition and one must recover evidence to analyze in order to create some sort of a profile, not merely detect a signal. It is also a matter of origin—whether the agent is natural or engineered, and to what degree in case of the latter. Even if a natural one, it may be perplexing: a known or unknown from some shadowy, dark and damp corner of a rainforest?

Human agency can be analyzed in generations of bioagents tampered/processed or simply acquired as occurring naturally and used as such. Before the Microbial Theory was conceived and the microbes detected, the processes available for (re)creating a disease or epidemic were well-known, established and followed. Some historic cases of targeted pestilence are exemplary on the subject, with the Black Death in Europe being a suitable example here, as a result of Mongolian biowarfare in Jaffa, which was blown out of proportion by travel and migration and also by chance. Once microorganisms were identified and manipulated for harvesting and dissemination, the first generation of bioagents came into being, with the Japanese biowarfare against the Chinese during 1930s being the most notorious example. From then on, different degrees of manipulation and tampering (e.g., enhanced Anthrax and Smallpox agents) were revealed at the turn of the millennium, all the way to engineered agents under the guise of gain-of-function studies and fully artificial agents through xenobiology and synthetic biology.

The second question is a combination of two really simple ones: the 'where' and 'when', that cover the spatio-temporal location (here, the term 'location' is used expansively and not restrictively in the literal, 3-D space context). This may sound natural, which it is, and straightforward, which it is not. The initial focus of an epidemic or any other biorisk is essential for predicting the dispersion pattern and thus containing it, before moving to decontamination and other steps, e.g., prioritized—and not uniform/horizontal—prophylaxis and protection of the exposed populations—human and others. Thus, an endemic origin and event, as opposed to an epidemic one, constitute a crucial character for the response to the event, in some degree by allowing a rough assessment of human agency or the spontaneous nature of a given outbreak.

The time of the onset is similarly important, as it provides the initial point to understand the temporal differences and thus the speed of any number of metrics. However, one very tricky issue is that the answers to the above pair of questions may not be unique; for example, the dispersion time and the onset of symptoms may vary considerably for agents with long incubation times, and this does not apply only to microbial agents. There are slow-acting biomolecular agents as well, and let us not forget about radiotoxins. This also affects the location footprint, whether the observed location of affected individuals is indeed the location of the release of the agent or its entry into the population (the former term would be used for perpetrated or possibly accidental events, and the latter for accidental or spontaneous ones).

The topography of the initiation of an event may be difficult to establish retrospectively due to the use of fomites and vectors, which may move an agent over long distances before its effects become detectable. This fact necessarily affects the temporal dimension; the transportation takes time and thus there is a temporal gap between the release/ingress/interface and the initiation or detectability of the effects. This is not necessarily a two-way occurrence: an agent may have a latent period and thus present detrimental effects at the very position of its release or ingress into the target community, population or ecosystem. *Some* drift may be expected by random causes, but this is not a constant. A time lapse does not necessarily mean a drastic relocation, although multiple events occurring in different locations do not necessarily mean some spatial revision either; other issues might be at play, including, but not limited to, multiple dispersion events. On the contrary, spatial divergence without a temporal difference almost unmistakably implies either a high dispersion event or different, concurrent dispersion events.

The "who" is the third question, revolving around the nature of the event; actually, whether it is spontaneous or perpetrated. There has been much effort to determine the nature of the origin of an event; the 2022 allegations of the Russians for bioattacks (committed or planned) in a manner compatible with natural microbiomics patterns shows, if nothing else, that this is an issue, or rather a parameter, taken well into consideration by biodefense experts *at least* in one country. The nature of the event is quintessential: perpetrated events tend to include different folds and incorporate counter-countermeasures to nullify or at least compromise the expected response meant to tackle an event. In some cases, knowing the nature of the event also allows a rather accurate projection of means and methods and thus a measure of the necessary commitment of resources, especially in unpopular or expensive measures such as quarantines/containment.

And then there is an external temporal dimension. Biosecurity efforts are clearly divided into prospective and retrospective phases. Further breakdown is also possible, but, suffice to say here, all measures, actions and procedures taken and in action before an incident, aiming to forestall it or to provide cognitive coverage (alarm, early warning), are proactive measures. All the procedures enacted after an incident has occurred and as a response to it are in the reactive realm. They are numerous and wildly different measures and actions, and many are very similar if not identical to proactive measures, simply scaled up in some manner and adapted for a more limited spatio-temporal setting.

Different systems have been proposed to assess the less straightforward parameters. If the weaponization of an agent is deemed highly probable, this would automatically make its detection as the cause of an event suspicious of human agency. Thus, formulas of risk assessment of an agent may be used for determining the causality of an event, at least indirectly—a legacy of the first few years of the 21st century. The weaponization potential can be assessed crudely, elaborately, or in an intermediate, more standardized manner. Such systems aim to assess the human-instigated, perpetrated risk factor and are thus integrated within the concept of biosecurity. The objective is a bit nefarious: the scores may be used (a) to reverse assess the spontaneity of an event, (b) to determine the ranking of possession of such an agent as a prospective WMD agent and thus initiate sanctions or other measures against a stakeholder, (c) to exclude trading of the agent and commodities potentially associated directly or indirectly with its acquisition and manipulation, and (d) for prioritization and security clearance of research on the agent.

Other scoring systems taking into consideration wildly different conditions—including biology (virulence), environment (population density, dispersion by air, stability in a given environment) and technology/policy (existence and availability of treatment options and facilities)—are used to sort agents in ascending order of accidental risk factor (biosafety levels) and thus authorize, or rather regulate their experimental use and, in the days to come, their use in biotechnological applications. Although the latter system refers to biosafety rather than biosecurity, a competent biosafety planning is quintessential for many biosecurity concerns, albeit not for all.

Biosecurity, as the risks evolve—or, more accurately, multiply in probable severity, possibility of outbreak and variety of threat agents is in dire need for recruiting any assistance from the respective sectors of -diverse- concerned parties. Networks and communications allow virtual specialists and better coordination of responses, while in the reactive setting. In a proactive setting, a better use of existing resources to achieve better (wider and in-depth) coverage of risk areas is achievable exactly due to such amenities. Advanced engineering solutions allow expanded sensor coverage for surveillance, both routine (proactive) and expedited (reactive). They are also focal in many aspects of tackling an event or crisis of the kind, especially in terms of decontamination, containment, quarantine (sterile delivery of supplies is essential in this case), evacuation and casualty management. Data mining in real time and correlation of the mined and livestreamed data resources are just as vital, with police and intelligence pipelines being fed into a biosecurity structure, either in an integrated way or *ad hoc*.

1

A (hi)story of Horror
Biosociomics as an Integrated Field to Critically Research the Occurrence of Biothreats throughout the Ages

M.E. Kambouris,[1,] Y. Manoussopoulos,[2] A. Velegraki[3] and G.P. Patrinos[4]*

Introduction

In the backdrop of multisectoral scientific endeavors, Science has been accepted within various domains of humanities. Owing to this, numerous issues have been resolved, with a more immediate and modern approach instead of the traditional, scholarly-only debate. Science demonstrates some prerogatives that are much more solid and evident than mere arguments, and the authority behind them, that governed humanities. It has been a "progress in the making".

---

[1] University of Patras, School of Health Sciences, Department of Pharmacy, Patras, Greece & The Golden Helix Foundation, London, United Kingdom.

[2] ELGO-Demeter, Plant Protection Division of Patras, Patras, Greece.
Email:inminz@gmail.com, ORCID iD: https://orcid.org/0000-0002-6065-7368

[3] Medical School, National and Kapodistrian University of Athens, Athens, Greece & Bioiatriki SA, Athens, Greece.
Email: aveleg@med.uoa.gr, ORCID iD: https://orcid.org/0000-0002-7605-0210

[4] University of Patras, School of Health Sciences, Department of Pharmacy, Patras, Greece & United Arab Emirates University, College of Medicine and Health Sciences, Department of Genetics and Genomics, & Zayed Center for Health Sciences, Al-Ain, Abu Dhabi, UAE.
Email: gpatrinos@upatras.gr, ORCID iD: https://orcid.org /0000-0002-0519-7776

* Corresponding author: mekambouris@yahoo.com, ORCID iD: https://orcid.org/0000-0002-3205-4797

Unfortunately, the two lines of thought are a world apart. The Humanities consider the science part simply a tool; following results from the scientific method, a pure scholarly debate and research within the field may be initiated—this is the interpretation of results of different scientific amenities, akin to carbon -and other ways of- dating. For a humanities researcher, the part of methodology is clear-cut and perhaps boring and mundane; so, science does a job to allow the real scholarly research to take place.

This point of view degrades the scientific constituent from Science to a mere technicality. The problem is that this is a somewhat restrictive and oversimplified view. Actually, the use of modern equipment is not entirely a matter of routine—it is a science in its own right—and the focal point is that the readings and results *are* actually interpretations of raw data. This is so much so as an application is innovative (a modern keyword extremely vague in its current use and thus highly lucrative) and has immense repercussions. Understanding this detail actually introduces a degree of uncertainty before the main phase of humanities research, that is, the argumentation—it is common knowledge in scientific research, with elaborate if not occasionally exaggerated efforts to curtail error and uncertainty. However, in humanities, the statistics are usually applied in the translation and not during the application of scientific techniques.

The object of this chapter is to discuss assets and liabilities, or rather advantages and disadvantages of the two lines of thought, and to suggest a method for integrating technology with social dimensions, and thus arrive at an improved, critical history of knowledge in biology and medicine. As the result of the above, a post-anthropocentric understanding of health and the need to consider the biological, social and political determinants of health synchronously will hopefully emerge (Özdemir 2020, 2021). To do so, apart from mere concepts, it is imperative to suggest possible ground rules for their cross-fertilization in the exploration of biomedical history in full view of modern technology, emerging challenges and established scholarship, and, which is infinitely more challenging, the conditions under which such rules may change, introducing an ingrained evolutionary potential.

The road so far

Even the most accurate and explicit historical records are faced with congenital bias: the recorder/narrator, even with the purest intent, had to please somebody to be granted the pass to immortality. Otherwise, the cognitive and supportive resources needed would have never been allocated to him. Thus, biased accounts and even more biased interpretations are widespread in the Humanities. Entire disciplines or subdisciplines are named after the precise nature and origin of such biases more subtly referred to as the 'lens of interpretation'. On the other hand, this is a part of the reason for developing excellent skills of argumentation. Humanities demand their disciples to be able to theorize, assume, suggest, test repeatedly, question in depth and advance with successive logical steps and suppositions; and to do so to an extent and depth unimaginable in Science, where data (and, currently, statistics and/or informatics) is the essence. The fabric of the scholarship of Humanities is considered speculation by the standards of Science.

Authorities and biases

The aforesaid is only a part of the story. When science explores a natural phenomenon, or even a social one, experimentation allows for proper controls to delineate the nature and true character of the query in both qualitative and quantitative terms, including the conditions, factors and parameters. This is a data-generation process— 'evidence generating' in more elegant parlance. Heavy processing by statistics and informatics ('dry lab') further enhances, and occasionally supplants, experimental tools with procedures usually reminiscent of simulations. The results are still open to interpretation and to manipulation—through the selection of conditions for the actual experimental procedure (wet lab or fieldwork), the informatics/algorithms and pipelines of dry lab and the levels of significance in statistics.

Enter reality. When dealing with an actual event, as is an epidemic, experimentation does not work. The events unfold in real time and uniquely, thus constituting evidence and feeding evidence-based analysis, while many factors and parameters are unknown. Here, the Uncertainty Principle can be expanded to imply that no two events are duplicates (even in experimental settings, much less in reality)—they differ in essence or time or both. Thus, accumulating data and projecting mathematical models is not very different from a high-order speculation with rules and arguments beyond the reach of non-experts. This is in stark contrast with the argumentation of humanities—which is approachable to anyone with standard linguistic skills and training in logic.

Thus, when approaching issues such as climate change, science becomes speculative. But the tools and know how of this trade, namely speculation, lie with humanities. As such, they are always plighted by bias, and have necessarily developed some dependable ways to check for it and, occasionally, rectify the issues discovered, subject to the will to do so, of course. What is even more important is that western science in general is not defraud of congenital bias and subjectivity. The issue of Authority is quintessential, followed by that of fashion. In research, there are tacit and less tacit non-institutional obligations in terms of conduct—bioethics is constitutional and a great step towards progress. On the other hand, there are issues with authority; academicism that stemmed from the bowels of the Catholic Church and in many cases its semi-feudal social footprint, especially the autonomy of its communities, is more than obvious and passes on the oligarchic concept of 'liberties' (euphemism for 'privileges') to the newer generation.

One must ponder upon statistics to see that authority-based, rather than evidence-based approaches are still with us. The concept of testing a hypothesis, formulating the null hypothesis and confirming or rejecting it, is still a matter of *authority*. It tests and controls it, but in principle accepts it. There is the authority of the assumption that is tested, instead of being imposed in many other cases (administration being one such case or factor). But a non-authority-based approach would have been 'agnostic'. The question is: "What happened?" and not "Was this an earthquake or a missile or Superman?"

Different times suggest different vogue currents. In the 1990s, medicine reluctantly embraced molecular biology and many prestigious journals rejected papers not using such—then novel—approaches or dendrograms, or which failed to submit results of Sanger sequencing to databases. Today, one has to engage in NGS and/or statistics to submit such papers or face rejection for failing in the latter criterion, irrespective of the actual need for doing so within the context of a specific research project. It is a convention of propriety and transgressors are encouraged to conform to have their work even considered.

Science of course needs rules for proper conduct: but it is one thing to judge (an editor's or reviewers' function is nothing short of passing a judgement) a method or conduct and the results and conclusions, and another to enforce one's own preferences on the means by exercising the power of passing a judgement. There are many stories on the deaths caused by physicians not washing their hands (Little 2020), as they considered it outrageous to accept that the physician could in any way harm the patient—a notion heard, read and projected nowadays for some forms of medicaments. The 'unique' way, the 'only' solution, the 'absolute' necessity to conform are all taken from the current and previous vocabulary of medical experts and remind of the unsavory preaching in a church.

Authority and its plights, well-established by the Social Sciences and Humanities, seem to be acceptable in Science, especially in biomedicine; and it is not a thing of today. A good example from history is the so-called 'Kehoe' problem—the leading scientific authority on environmental Lead (Pb) in the 1930s, whose findings came to determine an erroneous threshold limit for safe exposure to lead. This had massive negative effects on both environmental and public health sectors. The international community of science seems to operate as a guild, defined by specialty, and unable to resolve issues tackled by societies during the 19th century at the latest; entire fields of study, as mentioned earlier, are still governed by experts. Very few experts stemming from the Circle control the progress in their sector (the criterion of *recognition* in the CV of a scientist, a nominally vital issue) and the succession of the circle; church institutions are very similar in this reference. Assigning the title of 'top in [such] field' to an individual who has occupied the seat of power in a public scientific organization, foundation or institute for 30 or 40 years is unnerving—a stereotype reminiscent of clergy and aristocracy is less important than the notion that nobody has been considered functionally equal for 30 or 40 years. Is it a once-in-a-century/ lifetime event, like the new Buddha or Dalai Lama? Is it because the training and conscription realities fail to attract, produce and prepare equally, if not more, worthy scientists in successive generations? If that were the case, it would amount to total failure in Academia.

The History of Medicine is a very good example in this regard. It is the paradigmatic conversation of Biomedical Science and History, although not for a common purpose—while one of the two agents is the subject, the other is the object. History operates on, not with, Medicine. Moreover, the former is concerned with the approaches, progress, pitfalls, challenges and evolution of medicine as a practice and a science, not with the history of human (and others') health. However, it does provide a starting point. Paleontology follows suit; yet, even here (as is common whenever the prefix 'palaeo/paleo' is come across), one may suppose non-human objects and, very importantly, humans devoid of any contemporary or other historic descriptions and the double standard of a civilized life recording its context for collective and selective memories as a means of identification. The floor is to the scientist, his methods and findings.

Means and methods

Regarding the historical context, traditionally three axes were followed to study bioevents of the past (Cunha 2004)—the first axis includes accounts of varying extents, reliability and proficiency—the humanitarian dimension. The latter is far from homogenous and allows for two different approaches to the history of disease. These approaches are 'naturalist-realist' and 'historical-conceptual' (the terms are clearly amenable to improvement). The notion is that the former treats past disease experience on the basis of our present understanding and with the tools of both bioscience and humanities, whereas the latter places disease concepts within their historical contexts and thus keeps their aspects as by the protagonists of times past. This includes administrators, physicians and of course the affected masses of (not necessarily infected) populations (Lu and Yavetz 2021). It follows that the medical continuum of a culture at or during a specific period of time, conceptualized in integrative form as Iatromics (Hekim and Özdemir 2017), is a *very* humanities' issue.

Then, where applicable, comes the second axis—the (paleo-)microbiology dimension; this is usually understood in its clinical dimension—any trace or finding of specific microbiota or microbiomes, or their results and traces on remains and fossils. The latter infringes on paleopathology, where remains with pathological findings may be telling a story. Paleopathology specifically examines lesions found in remains to suggest damage characteristic of an ailment or pathogen. This deals with skeletal remains mostly; however, in mummifications, pathological findings of soft tissues, conditionally of course, and even microbiological findings may be expected.

Finally, the third axis is concerned with Epidemiological considerations, which apply mostly, but not entirely, to infectious diseases: cancer epidemiology, for example, may be very revealing. Of course, there is an issue here as well—the means by which epidemiology will get the *paleo-* prefix. For times within the same medical continuum, possibly since 17th century, this may be feasible, even with some limitations, mostly referring to the horizon of the science of the day. But for other eras or, to be precise, *any* other medical continuum, contemporary or not, this is somewhat challenging.

As a new era of destructive infectious diseases is emerging, our capability of fully recording and understanding the past may hold the key towards prognosis and possibly affect, if not even engineer, the future. It is futile, and perhaps wasteful, to document every flu outbreak of the last 4,000 years; but resolving near-extinction and Extinction-Level Events-ELEs and Global Catastrophic BioRisks-GCBRs (Palmer et al. 2017, Schoch-Spana et al. 2017) is important. This would suggest routines of change in clinical manifestations and other infection markers by existing pathogens and their ancestors, and could be correlated with paleogenomic data on human immunity mechanisms and traits. But without fully integrating literary sources, even myths, the functional dimension of the event/disease will always escape, and so will the accounts of damage as well, for soft tissues rarely survive and testimony is the only way available therefore. Even representational art becomes crucial to speculate the physical impacts of the pathogens and the ailments, although it tends to underscore deformities and disease phenotypes (Lu and Yavetz 2021).

Several subdisciplines of health sciences are used to decode issues and mysteries of the past within the context of humanities. Archaeological Chemistry is of marginal concern here, for it approaches the issues of Archaeology, not of Paleomedicine, and is applied to inanimate objects for identification, association or dating. The precise association of a metal to ores with local peculiarities is a very good example in this context; such data may well map both transportation and travel transactions, at least with an intermittent track. The identification of residues, given their chemical nature, may also aid in locating as well as understanding functions, know-how and practices. The matter of dating is pretty self-explanatory.

On the contrary, biomolecular archaeology (Hunter 2007), by definition, deals with both alive and dead objects. With the aid of molecular biology, it may identify the nature of textile remains (linen, cotton, silk) even spoiled to an extent that they are not recognizable by appearance and standard qualities (Kinti et al. 2012). The argumentation of dietary habits by analyzing skeletal remains is another aspect worth musing over.

Paleogenetics (Gaeta 2021) strives to identify the lineage of human and non-human populations beyond the living ancestral limits, whereas *paleogenomics* is the more inclusive and integrative spin-off therefrom (Demeure et al. 2019). Although the latter started as a new sector, it seems to be speeding towards an independent status, as a new discipline, with the multitude of research projects implemented throughout the globe, which elucidate population history and the migration patterns of current and/or historic populations.

Distinguishing the objective from the tool unambiguously is a sensitive topic. In Biomolecular Archaeology, the word 'biomolecular' denotes methodology and the object is archaeology ('archaeology' is concerned with animate and inanimate entities). The nature of the object varies with each specific project, but the biomolecular techniques are always present, thus justifying the title. On the contrary, in sectors such as paleopathology, paleomicrobiology and paleogenomics (Thèves et al. 2016, Demeure et al. 2019, Gaeta 2021), the prefix shows the nature of the object, and all conclusions on the methodological approaches remain conjectural and open. One can suppose that the standard methods of such sectors and disciplines can be used for their 'paleo-' iterations, subject to applicability. In this context, paleomicrobiology would initially indicate the ability to suggest the existence of specific microbiota by culturing them and identifying the spawn (usually if spores or other robust lifeforms have been formed and recovered or isolated), or if other tracks and signs have been conserved (enclosed in amber or otherwise encapsulated/fossilized, for instance). The imprint of calcium sheaths of Protoctista, for example, would suggest their presence even if the shell/sheath itself is destroyed along with the fully organic parts of the cell/organism. In this case, DNA tracks and signals are perfectly acceptable, subject to certain conditions of course. Thus, the *methodological* arm of paleogenomics/paleogenetics has been introduced (Demeure et al. 2019) to resolve queries of other subdisciplines rather than their own; paleogenomics may also effectively assist epidemiological considerations by producing a temporal perspective. Now, whether *paleometagenomics* would be a valid term, only time will tell.

A working example

The plague of Athens is the definition of GCBR (Palmer et al. 2017, Schoch-Spana et al. 2017, Kambouris et al. 2018), for it literally changed the course of history (Langmuir et al. 1985). It has attracted intense scholarly interest from both historians and physicians. A detailed account from a competent historian who was not only a contemporary, but also a survivor of the disease showcases (or, rather, its studies showcase) the possible pitfalls and limits of current processes regarding such matters (Langmuir et al. 1985, Cunha 2004).

One of the most detailed studies with excellent argumentation (Cunha 2004) appeared shortly before a supposed breakthrough. The latter; used paleogenomics, paleometagenomics actually (although not using the term), to detect possible pathogens and thus resulting in circumstantial evidence indicating towards *Salmonella enterica* var *typhi* as the most probable causative agent (Papagrigorakis et al. 2006) for outbursts of *typhoid fever.* The former study is an exemplary case of deduction and scholarship applied in the biomedical field, integrated with the analytical skill of humanities' experts. The arguments underlying such clinical considerations and diagnostic reasoning were of course based in paleomicrobiology and paleopathology (Cunha 2004), the norm before the advent of paleogenomics (Demeure et al. 2019). Now the latter can be applied to both paleomicrobiology and paleopathology and thus increases their spectrum; however, in the case of paleopathology, paleogenomics applies conditionally—mostly in cases of congenital diseases. Taking a sample of just three (groups of) papers on the subject, one may notice that a very thorough examination of literary, paleopathological, epidemiological and clinical dimensions led to a probable identification of the plague with measles caused by *Measles morbillivirus* (MeV), an RNA(-) virus (ICTV 2020)—a very important fact. It is not a perfect match, but the argumentation in favor of as well as against it is exemplary and convincing, although this solution is not one of the preferred ones among researchers who tackle this issue. The second approach (Papagrigorakis et al. 2006) made use of paleometagenomics through molecular amplification assays targeted to biomarker sequences of a number of possible causative agents. In this case, the approach is much more direct than the one previously mentioned (Cunha 2004) and has found a partial match only for *S. enterica* var. *typhi*. And hence, at this very point, starts the controversy.

The molecular approach did not search for possible pathogens, it sought *specific* pathogens in a binary fashion—yes/no for all seven of them in individualized assays. Only one of the seven produced a positive signal, which did not result in full confirmation when further tested. The sequence of the tested sample differed substantially from that of the respective reference sample, creating doubts of the validity of the classification achieved by phylogeny scores. Some strain of *Salmonella* could be a valid guess, but probably not one associated with typhoid fever (Shapiro et al. 2006) and, thus, little likely to be the cause of such lethal a plague. One may wonder what would have happened if the heterology or drift was at the sequences targeted by the primers used.

But, as is obvious, there are some more pressing issues. The first is that no RNA agents were included in the panel as there is no way such residue would have survived. So, this approach ignored the measles hypothesis from the outset. This argument may be extended a little further—to whether the panel was exhaustive, even regarding the DNA-genomed agents. Now, here the literary issue comes to play—in the matter of how exhaustive the panel was. It is clear that one would identify a number of higher probabilities from the billions of possible pathogens, using the literary account as a clinical and perhaps epidemiological compass since other approaches (paleopathology/paleomicrobiology) were of limited value. The very elaborate discussion that proposed a version of measles (Cunha 2004) and subsequently cast doubts over the advocates of *S. typhi* (Shapiro et al. 2006) used Occam's Razor efficiently to arrive at conclusions and took positive, negative as well as silent arguments into consideration. A third-party report (Littman 2009) suggesting and excluding measles from the list of possibilities did preciously little to counterargue against, but for epidemiology projections concerning unknown but alleged population, geographical and social parameters (an issue directly dependent on literary sources and their use and interpretation) and models depending on possibly inapplicable pathogens and transmission patterns. The epidemiological profile should rather be compiled from clinical and laboratory facts (syndromic surveillance), and not be used to surrogate in their absence. Epidemiology is not a given, but a query. In such cases, where possibly different or divergent strains have come in contact with a benign population and the event is unprecedented, exclusion seems rather ill-advised.

The matter of greater concern here is that the scientifically sound paleometagenomic research, seeking hard data with competent approaches, failed to take into consideration the possible case of co-existence/co-morbidity as well as the equally possible inclusion/exclusion indications of highly reliable contemporary literary sources (the History of Thucydides) providing an almost medical description of the clinical and epidemiological entity. In this context, some robust approaches of linguists and physicians, especially versed in the history of medicine (McSherry and Kilpatrick 1992), could well increase the value of the clinical/epidemiological report of Thucydides (Thuc II.48-52); all the three groups of papers reported here would have profited from this. Thucydides' words clearly imply an airborne pathogen since the people who attended the diseased individuals were the first to contract the ailment themselves (Thuc II.51,4-5). Although this does not exclude insect bites (Bazas 1994, Theodorides 1995), it does nothing to suggest them either, and this is not the same, in terms of argumentation. After all, Thucydides' narrative excludes very few things. Thus, any discussion of non-directly contagious pathogens should have been assigned a lower priority.

The vector of the epidemiological wave from the port of Piraeus to the city of Athens is equally important. It implicates two different, but not mutually exclusive, indications: the source of water (reservoirs in Piraeus, contrary to the running freshwater in the city) and the possibility of importing the ailment by commercial traffic. If the association of the Plague of Athens with the nearly contemporary ones of NE Africa and Asia (Thuc II.48,1) is valid (and this is a big "if"), searching relevant strata for remains to test by paleometagenomics would be a valid approach. Even then, some agents would be excluded due to technical limitations. But the populations of NE Africa, not being under siege, may have carried no markers of *S. typhi*, which is a very common finding in cases of poor hygiene and especially in crowded lodgings under siege (Thuc II.52). Instead, there may have been secondary (co-morbidity) or even no association (circumstantial finding) with the plague in question. In short, if one does not look for a plausible range of possibilities and limits oneself to the finite possibilities accessible by the selected methodology, the findings may be circumstantial and, if not filtered through other tests and assays, the conclusions may be of limited reliability, if not outright mistaken and/or biased. In this case, if one looks for *S. typhi* in a very condensed, hygienically challenged and unhealthy environment of a densely populated besieged city, it is highly probable to find and identify it. If not seeking measles, as the methodology denies such an ability, one cannot corroborate or discredit that possibility. And thus, by finding one of the limited agents one was searching for, it is possible to assign such circumstantial findings to the causal agency of a major event, throwing away what would be, in contemporary parlance, the testimony of the specialists; for typhoid, as we know it, is a poor match for Thucydides' account (Bellemore et al. 1994).

Such a testimony itself has certain limitations. It has been clearly suggested by Thucydides, a very competent, reliable and detailed source, that there was no hint of black rats or of any other vector (Langmuir et al. 1985, Cunha 2004, Fins 2020). One is entitled to question whether Thucydides would have reported any such event though. A symptom or sign, he would have had (McSherry 1995), for he was so meticulous in describing such matters that failing to do so would not have been a persuasive prospect. But rats and insects, these are another matter.

Linguists and scholars of humanitarian orientation are even more valuable for qualifying the historical context of the corps of evidence. One must consider the possibility that no rats, black or otherwise, were present, at least not among the pestilences of ancient Greece; neither were insects. This is somewhat difficult to accept, but it is a valid possibility and needs examination. For example, do the regions adjoining ancient Greece—Egypt, the Levant and Thrace—provide accounts of such incidents? If so, it is a bit weird to think that the Greek soil was virgin to such vermin. If not, one has an additional issue to ponder upon. Is there any other report in ancient Greek literature (tragedies, manuals on agriculture, or anything else), especially from the time of Thucydides, reporting such vermin? If rats and insects find no or 'few' mentions in the literature, a humanities' scholar would suppose that it is a vogue or convention of the era not to mention such disgusting creatures in highly aesthetic scholarly and literary works, This is not because such creatures are 'absent' or do not exact any degree of blood, sweat and tears, but because there is a tendency to scorn and overlook them. Another scholar would suggest that Apollo was the god of sudden death as well as of pestilence, using the surname Smintheus (after whom Smintheus.org, the database recording pathogens as per inclusion/exclusion in the select agents and toxins list of the US, is named). Consequently, some acknowledgement of disease and non-violent early deaths (Homer, The Iliad I.50-53), although tacit, is traceable.

The possibility that the word 'Smintheus' derives from 'sminthus', a word for rats (Burt 2006), underlines the connection and reminds of a *different* tradition, the Old Testament, where rats and vile creatures *are* mentioned (Köhler and Köhler 2003), as are snakes.

When one is met with so many uncertainties, assigning a causal status to an agent that does not really match a precise and concise clinical account because it is the only one out of seven tested agents that produced a partial DNA match may be a poor proof of guilt. And this has not even been properly tested by pure scientific standards. The dental pulp that was tested is a valid approach used elsewhere in paleomicrobiology/paleometagenomics, and had been analyzed with NGS nonetheless (Demeure et al. 2019), a much better proposal expected to detect multiple signals. But then comes the question:—was the dental pulp accessible by all pathogens of interest and could all of them be expected to survive there for so long (25 centuries)? Is the agent of measles among pathogens that may access the dental pulp and survive in there for two millennia?

One understands that in such cases, where the pioneer of modern medicine, Hippocrates, had failed to contain the pestilence (Thucydides account mentions nothing of the kind and suggest the plague raging for more than three years), it is very important, even vital, to know what the cause was. Was it a pathogen identical to the existing ones, one different from the current ones, or something virtually unimaginable? All the three cases lead to even more questions, infringing on social conditions, lifestyle, human immunity and possible hereditary traits affecting immunity and susceptibility. Being able to compare such historic data with different events in space and time, described in different languages and perhaps within a wholly different network of terms, procedures, practices and entities coming from another medical culture is of paramount importance. A combined history of pestilence outbreaks, epidemiology, human immunity and pathogen evolution can be manifested only by using software and linguistic tools imaginatively, rather than by bean-counting the sand or inventing new angles to reinterpret history. There are plenty of skills and sources; they must be simply put to better use.

An erroneous conclusion may result in fatal-or vital-consequences. It is the Echo Chamber Effect:—a view repeated and shielded from the acid test of criticism, questioning and scientific (or other, for that matter) challenging is actually amplified and gains importance, translatable to impact. After attempting a response to the said criticism (Papagrigorakis et al. 2007), the idea of typhoid fever being the culprit for the Plague of Athens expanded by incorporating anthropological, social, historical and political overtones by the reconstruction of one face of the sculls found intact in the mass grave; the reconstructed young female was named *Myrtis* and this entire episode became a major cultural event in Greece, suggesting that it was the face of an ancient Athenian female (Chickhistory 2010). More restrained voices (Archaeology News Network, 2010) suggested that it was the face of a *resident* of Athens, perhaps of a poor citizen family (women were not citizens themselves), but more probably a metic (resident alien) or, even more probably, a slave. The latter would explain the poor status, that is the lack of, ceremony, for slaves were disposed of in mass graves more freely than the citizenry, irrespective of the social status of the latter. The Athenian citizenry were the Master Race of the Eastern Mediterranean at the time and some ceremony and observance of ritual was expected for them and their womenfolk. Slaves, on the other hand would have died by the score due to congested and overpopulated conditions, lack of healthcare and lack of interest and forethought; they were disposed of unceremoniously.

The amplification of a nice, although scientifically unconvincing, story reached to the point of implicating issues of Bioterrorism (Papagrigorakis et al. 2013): the report of Thucydides, regarding a prophecy given to the Spartans—that the God (Apollo) would assist their cause if pursued rigorously, irrespective of their prayers or lack of them (Thuc I.118,3)—has been correctly interpreted as an indication of foul play. The ancient Athenians thought so themselves (Thuc II. 48,2) and foul play was very likely from the side of the enemy, and even more so from the Priesthood of Apollo. It certainly seems to involve a perpetrated and intentional use of a bioagent, but it is by no means an act of bioterrorism. It had been executed in a state of war and is thus an act of biological warfare, clandestine or not. But by no reading of modern parlance and terminology could it be considered "terrorism" (Kambouris 2021). This is a good example of an Echo chamber, using a valid scientific method to amplify the specific signal to higher volumes than the original output, and insulate it from outside "noise"—a very reliable method, but out of context here.

The immediate and mid-term prospects

Questioning the framing of a body of knowledge, before accepting its veracity and legitimacy, is a necessary new skillset in the 21st century. Previously described as "epistemic competence", it refers to the ability and willingness to examine the frames and framings in which knowledge is produced. It aims to integrate technology with social dimensions and produce a critical history of knowledge in biology and medicine (Özdemir et al. 2020, Özdemir 2021). Such a construct is not merely the moral duty of a scientist to the scientists of the past, it is more than a legacy or a trust meant for the ones of the future. It is a reappraisal of the past that may discover lost and hidden treasures. First, it changes 'facts' that are not facts but socially constructed surrogates of reality, serving a purpose rarely, if ever, altruistic, but often presented under the guise of altruism. At present, we are likely to be able to see only a selective version of progress—a range of works (artefacts, ideas, procedures and processes) that have survived through the forces of history irrespective of their scientific validity. Meticulous reappraisal of science as performed in the near and distant past may reveal breakthroughs of broad relevance that have not come to light because they were suppressed by the local forces of their times, as well as by erroneous paths and ways that remained unchallenged and spiked the course of history.

The Black Death may be a suitable example of this case. Plague outbursts and epidemics are known and well substantiated (Zietz and Dunkelberg 2004, Demeure et al. 2019). Paleogenomics also allowed for a phylogenic and evolutionary chart of *Yersinia pestis* since its emergence from *Yersinia pseudotuberculosis*, an enteropathogen that evolved by genome reduction and gene gain (Demeure et al. 2019). Still, although a molecular history profile of the pathogen is available (Drancourt and Raoult 2016), the impact, massiveness and epidemiology of the *Y. pestis* plague (especially the bubonic plague) is far from a perfect match. Brilliant mental constructs and innovative ideas have been proposed to this end, and many of them are not bereft of merit, such as the development and evolution of novel vectoring possibly allowing human-to-human vector-borne transmission by human ectoparasites/insects (Dean et al. 2018), and not through black rat fleas (Cunha 2004, Dean et al. 2018, Demeure et al. 2019). Despite that, although a very unpopular opinion, it is possible that another pathogen, a wholly different agent that could progress much faster than rats and humans of the time, meaning a broadly airborne pathogen, should be sought for (Scott and Duncan 2001), without rejecting the *Y. pestis* implication and presence, but rather as comorbidity than as the sole cause. This view has very few supporters, but the beaked masks used at the time can be understood as a form of protection from something conditionally airborne (perhaps droplets) and not insect-borne or vector-borne in general, nor something primarily communicated by fomites (MacKenzie 2001), although such secondary transmission is far from implausible, as is the case with COVID-19.

Quo vadis?

Paleomicrobiology and Paleopathology are useful and well-known terms and concepts (Cunha 2004), and there is no reason not to expand the family: paleogenomics should be used whenever the discipline is practiced upon relic material, from graves or other natural repositories of remains, including fossils (Fox 2018). The prefix "paleo-" indicates work with material relics recovered and the need to tackle all assorted methodological difficulties (including, but not limited to classification and dating), but not any literary input of contemporary or non-contemporary sources to (re)create the context; it may refer to humans before the invention of written or oral accounts, or wildlife. A term indicating the availability of literary source should be defined. The Greek archaeo is much more appealing and ubiquitous as a prefix than the English "ancient"—consider "archaeology"—but the naming of some prokaryota as *Archaea* makes the idea unworkable. The easy solution—to add "archae-" before everything (genomics, iatromics, infectiomics, microbiomics)—is simple and straightforward but not appealing. The concept of biomolecular archaeology is valid; the term still lacks in the inclusiveness of OMICS sciences and, more importantly, implies the resolution of archaeological matters, such as the pedigree of remains, the homogeneity of populations, migration events, biological identification of findings and so on. The resolution of biological incidents, in this case medical ones, is of paramount importance. Non-medical cases are also of vital interest: identifying the agents and course and signs of other pestilence such as famines like the Great Hunger of Ireland, 1845–52 (Geber 2014) or of extinction-level events of a number of species may be very illustrative of environmental and also of social perils; massive loss of food sources cause social unrest, disorder, wars and widespread deaths by hunger; the victim count in such events may be in the order of millions.

A better, more integrative, and less 'techno-governed' and 'techno-restricted' concept of studying massive events of health casualties in the past is the need of the hour. This would involve pathogens and/or toxins, or events of massive impact as is the death of sovereigns by such agents (e.g., Tamerlan). The authors, pondering upon issues previously mentioned regarding the rules of conduct and the '*cell to society*' aspect of bioevents and phenomena (Özdemir 2021) propose the term *Biosociomics* as an inclusive term for the holistic, systematic and integrative research on bioevents entailing literary or other (e.g., representational) human testimonies on the said events; this has previously been described (rather in an introductory form) through various phrases, including 'ancient DNA literature' (Shapiro et al. 2006) and '...historic genomic, archeologic data' (Namouchi et al. 2018). The focus herein would be to expertly use modern technological and other scientific amenities to corroborate, and not simply reject, literary sources, preferably after a critical examination of their validity. This opens the stage for true multidisciplinary research, as historians, philologists, etc., are uniquely qualified to determine the validity of a literary source and to interpret it as well.

Assigning a medical culture element, transcending time through testimony (representational, written or spoken/oral) brings the study into the realm of Iatromics, as the latter were coined only a few years ago (Hekim and Özdemir 2017). This may facilitate inclusive, integrated research on such issues. Different Iatromics traditions should be conformed to a unique, wide-access megadatabase. Both linguists and scientists should be hired to translate and align, or rather plot such Iatromic/medical spheres of knowledge in order to enhance the perspective by exploring the paleomedicinal view of the history of medicine. Both ancient Greek and Oriental (especially Chinese) medical practices have survived in corpuses of extensive scientific literature that may become handy in recognizing reemerging threats in the form of ailments. The miasmatic qi of the Chinese (Lu and Yavetz 2021) lacks an understanding of microbial ailments as microbiology had not been invented/discovered at the time, but it still does afford valid knowledge and perception of geoepidemiology (Gkantouna et al. 2015), as local conditions are key for the prevalence of microbial disease in epidemic waves and tend to retain their morbid character for many years, occasionally even millennia (Lu and Yavetz 2021), unless environmental or other major changes occur (drainage of stale waters for instance). The modern fascination with pandemics and pathogens dispersed by trade, travel and migration intercontinentally tends to forget that a microbial disease was an endemic plight for most of the human history, from malaria to plagues (Raman et al. 2020, Lu and Yavetz 2021).

It is equally important to tap into resources of pharmaceutical interest. Plants were the mainstay in Chinese thought (Lu and Yavetz 2021); in the West, it was the Greek Dioscorides Pedanius, a military surgeon of the Roman Army in the 1st century CE, who compiled a very extensive guide to medicinal plants (*De materia medica*). The respective therapeutic herbal tradition was much more ancient though—pre-dating the dawn of the 1st millennium BCE, as evident from Homeric testimony (Homer, the Iliad, XI 841-7). However, animal products are also included (MacKinney 1946), along with ores/minerals, especially in oriental *materia medica* (Parker 1915), although the Greeks also used crystals, as evident in the Orphics, Lithica (Kostov 2008); this could be understood as a primitive effort towards therapeutical radiomics (*sensu lato*), as it dealt with assigning specific wavelengths (in a proportional manner) to ailments. Empirical practices exiled to mystification and occult or even lore may become very relevant in times of failing R&D budgets.

Bibliography

Archaeology News Network. (2010). The face of an 11 year old girl from Classical Athens, https://archaeologynewsnetwork.blogspot.com/2010/04/face-of-11-year-old-girl-from-classical.html. Last accessed: Mar 22 2022.

Bazas, T. (1994). The plague of Athens. Journal of the Royal Society of Medicine, 87(12): 755.

Bellemore, J. et al. (1994). Plague of Athens-fungal poison? Journal of the History of Medicine and Allied Sciences, 49(4): 521–545. doi: 10.1093/JHMAS/49.4.521.

Burt, J. (2006). Rat. London: Reaktion Books.

Chick History. (2010). Mystery of Myrtis: Ancient Athenian Girl Turned Global Ambassador, https://chickhistory.org/2010/10/01/mystery-of-myrtis-part-1-ancient-athenian-girl-turned-global-ambassador/Last accessed: Mar 22 2022.

Cunha, B.A. (2004). The cause of the plague of Athens: Plague, typhoid, typhus, smallpox, or measles? Infectious Disease Clinics of North America, 18(1): 29–43. doi: 10.1016/S0891-5520(03)00100-4.

Dean, K. et al. (2018). Human ectoparasites and the spread of plague in Europe during the Second Pandemic. Proceedings of the National Academy of Sciences of the United States of America, 115(6): 1304–1309. doi: 10.1073/PNAS.1715640115.

Demeure, C. et al. (2019). *Yersinia pestis* and plague: An updated view on evolution, virulence determinants, immune subversion, vaccination, and diagnostics. Genes and Immunity, 20(5): 357–370. doi: 10.1038/S41435-019-0065-0.

Drancourt, M. and Raoult, D. (2016). Molecular history of plague. Clinical microbiology and infection : the official publication of the European Society of Clinical Microbiology and Infectious Diseases, 22(11): 911–915. doi: 10.1016/J.CMI.2016.08.031.

Fins, J. (2020). Pandemics, protocols, and the plague of athens: Insights from thucydides. The Hastings Center Report, 50(3): 50–53. doi: 10.1002/HAST.1132.

Gaeta, R. (2021). Ancient DNA and paleogenetics: Risks and potentiality. Pathologica, 113(2): 141–146. doi: 10.32074/1591-951X-146.

Geber, J. (2014). Skeletal manifestations of stress in child victims of the Great Irish Famine (1845–1852): prevalence of enamel hypoplasia, Harris lines, and growth retardation. American Journal of Physical Anthropology, 155(1): 149–161. doi: 10.1002/AJPA.22567.

Gkantouna, V.A. et al. (2015). Introducing dAUTObase: A first step towards the global scale geoepidemiology of autoimmune syndromes and diseases. Bioinformatics, 31(4): 581–6. doi: 10.1093/bioinformatics/btu690.

Hekim, N. and Özdemir, V. (2017). A general theory for "Post" systems biology: Iatromics and the Environtome. OMICS : A Journal of Integrative Biology, 21(7): 359–360. doi: 10.1089/OMI.2017.0080.

Hunter, P. (2007). Dig this. Biomolecular archaeology provides new insights into past civilizations, cultures and practices. EMBO Rep, 8(3): 215–7. doi: 10.1038/sj.embor.7400923.

ICTV. (2000). Taxonomy History https://talk.ictvonline.org/taxonomy/p/taxonomy-history?taxnode_id=20181616.

Kambouris, M.E. et al. (2018). Rebooting bioresilience: A multi-OMICS approach to tackle global catastrophic biological risks and next-generation biothreats. OMICS A Journal of Integrative Biology, 22(1): 35–51. doi: 10.1089/omi.2017.0185.

Kambouris, M.E. (2021). Exploring the concepts: Biosecurity, biodefence and biovigilance. *In*: Kambouris, M.E. (ed.). Genomics in Biosecurity. 1st edn. Elsevier Academic Press.

Kinti, M. et al. (2012). SEM and FTIR analyses combined with sequence-based direct identification of deterioration-associated fungi enhances identification of excavated 5th c BC palaiotextile samples. Mycoses, 55(4): P.483.

Köhler, W. and Köhler, M. (2003). Plague and rats, the "plague of the Philistines", and: what did our ancestors know about the role of rats in plague. International Journal of Medical Microbiology, 293(5): 333–340. doi: 10.1078/1438-4221-00273.

Kostov, R. (2008). Orphic lithica as a source of late antiquity mineralogical knowledge. Annual of the University of Mining and Geology "St. Ivan Rilski", 51(1): 109–115.

Langmuir, A. et al. (1985). The Thucydides syndrome. A new hypothesis for the cause of the plague of Athens. The New England Journal of Medicine, 313(16): 1027–1030. doi: 10.1056/NEJM198510173131618.

Little, B. (2020). It took surprisingly long for doctors to figure out the benefits of hand washing. History. Mar 6 https://www.history.com/news/hand-washing-disease-infection.

Littman, R. (2009). The plague of Athens: epidemiology and paleopathology. The Mount Sinai Journal of Medicine, 76(5): 456–467. doi: 10.1002/MSJ.20137.

Lu, D. and Yavetz, Z. (2021). History of epidemics in China: Some reflections on the role of animals. Asian Medicine. Brill, 16(1): 137–152. doi: 10.1163/15734218-12341487.

MacKenzie, D. (2001). Did bubonic plague really cause the Black Death? | New Scientist. Available at: https://www.newscientist.com/article/mg17223184-000-did-bubonic-plague-really-cause-the-black-death/(Accessed: 14 March 2022).

MacKinney, L.C. (1946). Animal substances in materia medica A STUDY IN THE PERSISTENCE OF THE PRIMITIVE. Journal of the History of Medicine and Allied Science, 1(1): 149–170.

McSherry, J. and Kilpatrick, R. (1992). The plague of Athens. Journal of the Royal Society of Medicine, 85(11): 713.

McSherry, J. (1995). The plague of Athens. Journal of the Royal Society of Medicine, 88(4): 240.

Namouchi, A. et al. (2018). Integrative approach using *Yersinia pestis* genomes to revisit the historical landscape of plague during the Medieval Period. Proceedings of the National Academy of Sciences of the United States of America, 115(50): E11790–E11797. doi: 10.1073/PNAS.1812865115.

Özdemir, V. et al. (2020). COVID-19 health technology governance, epistemic competence, and the future of knowledge in an uncertain World. OMICS : A Journal of Integrative Biology, 24(8): 451–453. doi: 10.1089/OMI.2020.0088.

Özdemir, V. (2020). "One Nature": A new vocabulary and frame for governance innovation in post-COVID-19 planetary health. OMICS : A Journal of Integrative Biology, 24(11): 645–648. doi: 10.1089/OMI.2020.0169.

Özdemir, V. (2021). From the Editor's Desk: Systems Science 2010–2020, and Post-COVID-19. OMICS : A Journal of Integrative Biology, 25(2): 73–75. doi: 10.1089/OMI.2021.0002.

Palmer, M. et al. (2017). On defining global catastrophic biological risks. Health Security, 15(4): 347–348. doi: 10.1089/HS.2017.0057.

Papagrigorakis, M. et al. (2013). The plague of Athens: an ancient act of bioterrorism? Biosecurity and Bioterrorism : Biodefense Strategy, Practice, and Science, 11(3): 228–229. doi: 10.1089/BSP.2013.0057.

Papagrigorakis, M.J. et al. (2006). DNA examination of ancient dental pulp incriminates typhoid fever as a probable cause of the Plague of Athens. International Journal of Infectious Diseases, 10(3): 206–214. doi: 10.1016/J.IJID.2005.09.001.

Papagrigorakis, M. et al. (2007). Ancient typhoid epidemic reveals possible ancestral strain of Salmonella enterica serovar Typhi. Infection, genetics and evolution : Journal of Molecular Epidemiology and Evolutionary Genetics in Infectious Diseases, 7(1): 126–127. doi: 10.1016/J.MEEGID.2006.04.006.

Parker, L.A. (1915). A brief history of materia medica. The American Journal of Nursing. JSTOR, 15(8): 650–653. doi: 10.2307/3404151.

Raman, J. et al. (2020). High levels of imported asymptomatic malaria but limited local transmission in KwaZulu-Natal, a South African malaria-endemic province nearing malaria elimination. Malaria Journal. BioMed Central, 19(1). doi: 10.1186/S12936-020-03227-3.

Schoch-Spana, M. et al. (2017). Global catastrophic biological risks: Toward a working definition. Health Security, 15(4): 323–328. doi: 10.1089/hs.2017.0038.

Scott, S. and Duncan, C. (2001). Biology of Plagues. Cambridge: Cambridge University Press.

Shapiro, B. et al. (2006). No proof that typhoid caused the Plague of Athens (a reply to Papagrigorakis et al.). International Journal of Infectious Diseases : IJID : official Publication of the International Society for Infectious Diseases, 10(4): 334–335. doi: 10.1016/J.IJID.2006.02.006.

Theodorides, J. (1995). The plague of Athens. Journal of the Royal Society of Medicine, 88(6): 363.

Thèves, C. et al. (2016). History of smallpox and its spread in human populations. Microbiol Spectr, 4(4): PoH-0004-2014. doi: 10.1128/microbiolspec.PoH-0004-2014. 27726788.

Zietz, B.P. and Dunkelberg, H. (2004). The history of the plague and the research on the causative agent *Yersinia pestis*. International Journal of Hygiene and Environmental Health, 207(2): 165–178. doi: 10.1078/1438-4639-00259.

2

Agrosecurity
Integrating the Containment of Agroterrorism, Promotion of Bioeconomy and Protection of the Public Health

Yiannis Manoussopoulos,[1] *Aristea Velegraki,*[2]
Marianna Manoussopoulou[3] *and Manousos E. Kambouris*[4,*]

Introduction

When biosecurity is concerned, the idea of environment, with the operational aspect of the term, can be understood as a triplet of extremely different though interacting entities. The first is the human community in the public health setup and thus dealing mostly with the human species (in the urban environment mostly, but not exclusively), with the exception of a small number of domesticated animal species for company (pets) or for recreational purposes (zoos, aquariums, exhibitions, circuses, etc.) and ornamental plants as in cities and towns (pavements, parks, etc.) or in-house (flower pots, window boxes, yards, gardens, etc.). A shadow population of pests, such as

[1] ELGO-Demeter, Plant Protection Division of Patras, Patras, Greece.
Email: inminz@gmail.com, ORCID iD: https://orcid.org/0000-0002-6065-7368
[2] Medical School, National and Kapodistrian University of Athens, Athens, Greece & Bioiatriki SA, Athens, Greece.
Email: aveleg@med.uoa.gr, ORCID iD: https://orcid.org/0000-0002-7605-0210
[3] ELGO-Demeter, Plant Protection Division of Patras, Patras, Greece; and University of Padua, Department of Agronomy, Food, Natural Resources, Animals and Environment, Italy.
Email: mariannamasopoul@gmail.com
[4] University of Patras, School of Health Sciences, Department of Pharmacy, Patras, Greece & The Golden Helix Foundation, London, United Kingdom.
* Corresponding author: mekambouris@yahoo.com, ORCID iD: https://orcid.org/0000-0002-3205-4797

insects, cockroaches and rats also thrive in this environment; these interactions are more or less predictable, although the actions needed always pose a great concern.

The Environment at large is the opposite; divided into Wildlife and Agriculture, it is characterized by the scarcity of the human subject, with the well-known physiological, immunological and other biochemical characteristics studied by generations of physicians. The Environment includes populations very different from those mentioned above. Wildlife has high or low numbers of extremely diverse populations, while Agriculture—from orchards and farm animals in small numbers or in flocks, to plantations massive enough to be called *farm factories*, along with beehives or fishery—has highly homogenous and generally speaking dense populations, occasionally of very little interspecific genetic diversity as clonal exploitations are a widespread tendency.

There is also the rural context, somewhere at the middle, with diverse characteristics and metrics. In nature, it is an environmental setup, with all the intricacies of the latter, usually but not necessarily less genetically homogenous than agriculture, at least in the modern intensive agricultural context. But there are dispersed enclaves of solid human populations, relatively small but highly dispersed and cohesive. This creates an awkward fusion: the political sensitivity and priority of the urban setting with difficulties of the environment in terms of host range, potential pathogen variety and microbiome diversity. The last issue is critical. Environments created by settled human communities house complex microbiomes (Kambouris and Velegraki 2020, Velegraki and Zerva 2020), mostly saprobiotic but also parasitic to quite an extent. Parasitism usually features steady and narrow host selection, but more generic trends arise, especially with opportunistic pathogens which usually double as saprobiota. In many cases the pathogenicity is not a solid trait but rather a diversion from the usual, rather harmonious, co-existence in mutualism or, more often, commensalism (see Chapter 5).

Agrosecurity and Agroterrorism: concepts and timelines

Agrosecurity as a term came to prominence in the 1990s (DeOtte 2007), as a response to the agroterrorism threat (Gyles 2010) which was growing as a divergent discipline of bioterrorism back in the day. The different trade wars in the post-Cold War era and the acute issue of international drug trafficking and commerce (re)introduced it as a concern and as a means. Believed to be a method of what is now termed Hybrid Warfare, it could afford leverage in international affairs, especially to non-state players, against areas, groups and whole countries—some of the latter overly focusing their economic activity into the primary sector. Some countries could not diversify their economies, some others needed such focus to sustain their population and still others kept such focus because there was a lucrative export market for their produce. As a result, malefactors had it easy. Not sanctified as human life and health, much less guarded against perpetrators, with conditions helpful in the spreading of any disease in all sorts of exploitations especially intensive farming (planting and breeding), the Agro sector was a tempting, soft target with possibly great repercussions and asymmetrical impact as to the effort and risk of the perpetrator. A usually forgotten issue on the subject is that the targeting of the agro sector was an insurance policy of highly developed countries, warranting regular imports from abroad to sustain their population which was working largely in high-tech industries, to guard against the leverage that low-end economies enjoyed by virtue of control on such supplies. This latter concern led highly developed countries, such as Switzerland, to maintain a sufficient and thriving agro sector (Bötsch 2004, Unknown 2017), even at a significant cost, not that much for export purposes as for home use during distress.

For the generations grown in the western world, in thriving societies with an abundance of food supply (but NOT relevant production), agrosecurity was a rather marginal issue. It was referring to the interests of farmers—usually heavily subsidized (Monke 2004, Knowles et al. 2005, Pravecek et al. 2006, Unknown 2017). The deliberate dimension that multiplied the severity of the potato late blight and the resulting Great Famine of Ireland during 1845–1849 (Fraser 2003) is far less direct and obvious than the intentional starvation policies discussed and occasionally enacted in the 19th and 20th centuries in Europe and the Americas (Graziosi 2004, Claus 2020). But given that at least since 2008 (Tenenbaum 2008) the specter of famine has re-emerged and the supply chains remain disrupted after the COVID-19 shock (Pujawan and Bah 2021), global trade malfunctions and cargo ship-traffic issues, agrosecurity is no more an issue limited to the income and welfare of farmers and their ability and prerogative to live the dream and prosper. It has rather become a vital issue for securing sufficiency of supplies by affected communities. Moreover, due to the unorthodox development allowed or encouraged by globalization, communities very distant from the directly affected agricultural exploitations are threatened and concerned as their outsourced supply is endangered, as shown in 2022 with the Russo-Ukrainian war.

Agrosecurity and Agroterrorism are NOT merely an outcrop of Biosecurity and Bioterrorism. First, although it might be considered erroneous, there is not a direct counterpoart of biowarfare in the "agro-" context; very few speak of agrowarfare or agricultural biowarfare (Ban 2000, Olsen 2003, Ryan 2018, Kaur 2019). The latter should have been included indeed: the Allies were planning on using such approaches to starve Germany in WW II, by processes including but not limited to "Operation Vegetarian" (Rosie 2001, Kageyama 2021); the Germans started implementing similar measures against the Soviets, such as the "Hunger Plan" (Tooze 2006). The US did so twice; the first was in the Sioux wars, by slaughtering the buffaloes (Phippen 2016), the main food source of the tribes (it is a detail of minimal importance that those buffaloes were wild and not bred, for the economy of the Sioux nation had formed around hunting as a standard and not occasional process and activity); the other instance was the mass destruction of fishery nets by the US Underwater Demolition Teams in Korea so as to starve the pro-Communist population (Unknown 2022). Famines did ensue in both the cases. The issue became focal in the 1990s as the US was contemplating (and perhaps did use) bioagents to destroy crops of marijuana plants in Latin America (Rogers et al. 1999). The use of such agents in the territories of foreign states with which there was no state of war declared as such was extremely controversial.

The first issue is the definition of state-sponsored or conducted terrorism (or undeclared war). The niceties of dependent governments *asking* for assistance was obviously a pretext and did not hold water in many cases.

The second issue was the violation, at least in spirit, of the treaties for ban on bioweapons. Targeting non-human entities, especially ones detrimental to human health and life, was a *mantra* to bypass the issue, as the aforementioned spirit was set in the BioWeapons Convention (BWC). This *was* holding water, at least before concepts of animals' rights and non-human life in general emerged. Such principles would not accept precedence of human interests, dubious in this case, against mass destruction of lifeforms showing no spontaneous aggressiveness. Plainly put, narcotics was a problem of humans and using bioweapons against plants that were the original source, the raw materials for producing the said drugs, had to be avoided. Humans could shoot it out among themselves and leave the plants alone.

Another interesting issue is that agrosecurity and agroterrorism are not *subcases* of biosecurity and bioterrorism, respectively, and nor of biocrime, by any interpretation (see Chapter 10 and Introduction). The latter is correctly exempt as an agrothreat always has a massive impact. Although 'crime', 'terrorism' and 'warfare' are terms used as policy dictates and largely interchangeably, the notion of biocrime usually follows that of conventional crime, meaning small-scale events.

Regarding the association of the *agro-* entities with their *bio-* equivalents, or rather with their respective bio- numbers, the most important differentiation is that biothreats are not the only causative factor for agroterrorism (and thus the sole concern for consideration by agrosecurity), but only a part. Contrary to bioterrorism where the means give the name (the bioagents), the *target* names the faculty in agroterrorism: it is the terrorism against the agro sector as opposed to the terrorism *using* bioagents. Consequently, agrosecurity responds to threats targeting the agro sector, while biosecurity responds to threats posed by bioagents. As a result, a microorganism or a metabolite that is not poisonous for lifeforms but destroys an amenity, such as cables (as in wired telecommunications or electric apparatuses) or rubber (as in tyres), is a biothreat and an issue of biosecurity. Conversely, the core of agrosecurity includes the use of inorganic chemicals to spike soil in order to make it infertile (Owens 2001), or the use of radioactive waste to contaminate supplies by entering the food chain and thus rendering entire stretches of land barren and/or turning them into actual health hazards. It also includes the use of synthetic pesticides to destroy an actual crop and even the use of incendiaries to destroy crops, despite no bioagent being involved. Agrosecurity and biosecurity share important common elements, but neither is a part of the other.

Agrosecurity and agroterrorism: Prospects and realities

It is obvious that a prime concern in agrosecurity is the plant or animal produce; qualitatively or quantitatively diminished production, or its pause, may directly or indirectly cause famine and, more probably, economic loss and far-reaching disruptive effects—as was obvious with the disruptive effects of the COVID-19 pandemic in the global supply networks resulting in a marked drop of income for producers, even without any serious or actual agroterrorism activity. The disruptive effects impacted the supply chains, and through them the agro sector, resulting in lower production, shortages and massive income loss at both the ends of the chain— producers and consumers. But there are many other aspects in the threat. There are non-edible products that are vital for some economies: exportable amenities, industrial (such as cotton) or luxury (such as silk), may have profound economic effect therefore. For some cultures, medicinal plants are the only available option as modern medicine is inaccessible; hence, they center explicitly around Traditional, Alternative and Complementary Medicines-TACM (Kramlich 2014); it may also be an important issue for mainstream pharmaceuticals, especially for biological and low footprint production setups as projected in some states in contrast to highly polluting chemical synthesis. This trait is expected to gain momentum with biopharmaceuticals even more; plant essences and toxins may be found to be exploitable as sustainable antimicrobials.

Biofuel and at a later point bioelectricity are among the amenities that may come in fashion and thus be threatened by agrothreats. Even low-level and temporary degradation of electricity supply may cause enormous problems in medical or other sectors (Özdemir 2018, 2021), as well as in Big Data communication and electronic control and function optimization of appliances and devices, especially in the era of the Internet-of-Things (IoT). Finally, there, is the sector of high-tech projects, the production of body armor from spider silk for instance (Woody 2020), an enabler in the coming decades for projecting lethal and non-lethal power beyond state borders for any concern having such technology and sufficient productive capacity. If forestry and open field culturing of microbiota (i.e., mushrooms) are counted in the agricultural sector and not in the industrial sector, further applications can be identified and thus targeted for derailment by agroterrorism (and identified as concerns for agrosecurity), as are biorestoration and bioremediation of polluted soils or water bodies (Satijn and de Boks 1988, Verma and Sharma 2017, Janssen and Stucki 2020). The same applies to surface mining-ore enrichment and *in situ* processing (Marrero et al. 2015, Cockell et al. 2020). In the near term isolated areas and barren lands may be reclaimed and exploited in a context of extensive (rather than intensive) exploitation (Singh et al. 2020, Lau et al. 2022, Suman et al. 2022) and they would pose an asymmetric challenge in agrosecurity, given the novel bioengineered nature of the agents involved. In general, the agrosecurity of Genetically Modified Organisms- GMOs is a vast and very complicated chapter of biosecurity, since GMOs used occasionally on a larger scale could themselves pose agrosecurity risks on different accounts: from being sources of genetic pollution right up to hostile habitat takeover (Steinhäuser 2001, Bawa and Anilakumar 2013, Thomas and De Tavernier 2017).

The genetic pollution argument is decades old and has not yet been convincingly resolved, for the economics of such issues tend to reinforce the notions of the critics that high volumes of novel sequences would become available for fostering at the same time as unknown recombinations with native exogenomes in different microbiomes and ecosystems. Simultaneously, recombinations of same and similar species through viral interactions would also be possible. In short, similar and dissimilar taxa would be exposed to the interactions of genetic elements. These may be random sequences, possibly produced by spontaneous DNA degradation or, alternatively, whole genes and regulatory elements uptaken and combined, rearranged, modified and finally recombined with other genomic elements in a multitude of dissimilar recipients.

The hostile habitat takeover, possibly described with many more politically correct figures of speech, implies the introduction of an alien species resulting in the gradual or abrupt eradication of the original species. GMOs may result in functional toxicity against similar, unmodified organisms by simply having inserted a toxin/antidote gene system of any degree of sophistication in their genome. Thus, the soil may be rendered hostile and unusable for the original, unmodified species that do not have the genetic code for neutralizing or subverting the toxin. The toxin may be produced by the GMO or contained in appropriate pesticides and herbicides used in combination with the GMO (Anderson et al. 2019, Seralini 2020).

However, agrosecurity goes further than the immediate output/product. Disruptive effects may have resounding impact; the concept of waste disposal as a high-sustainability procedure in the context of circular economy (Adami and Schiavon 2021) may well be a risk factor. If not optimally managed, waste accumulation, especially in dispersed contexts, may cause epidemics and this is manifested whenever strikes or circulation disruption create towers of garbage in Mega-cities (Wankhede and Wanjari 2021). Deregulating the biological basis of this system would cause public health risks and perhaps deterioration of the environment by pollution.

Though the insertion of pathogens in the urban environment is the vital and usually unrecognized issue. By itself, the urban environment is not very permissive for microbiota to thrive, spread and evolve, compared to the ones already hosted, given the well-managed waste disposal and produce distribution. For the reasons mentioned above, the agro sector is a very permissive and host-rich environment for propagation and evolution of microbiota; it thus follows that reservoirs are located there, and the massive transportation of organic and inorganic matter from rural and agrarian environments to the urban ones (Kambouris et al. 2018) indicates that many microbiota would find their way and make the trip to the urban world. This can be done using either alternative and/or intermediate hosts or fomites as vectors. Rats and insects are the usual vectors for a range of microbiota, especially in rural environments, while direct transportation of airborne particles is a cause of allergies and respiratory conditions, as are the conidia of many opportunistically pathogenic mycelial fungi (Kurup et al. 2000, Li et al. 2019). It is obvious that with the expanded host range come the most important risk factors in the aspect of public health risks, whence the pathogens are inbound from the natural to the technidal environment (Kambouris et al. 2020a)—rural or urban.

The vast expanse, diversity and high density of hosts in the agricultural sector and secondarily in wild environments make the conventional procedures applied in public health utterly untenable. The surveillance of large areas requires round-the-clock, affordable and dense surveillance modalities for signs of risk factors since, contrary to humans, other hosts may not be able to utter comprehensible distress signals to assist in understanding the problem. The seer expanse suggests unmanned systems (drones) for monitoring and intervention. Aerial vehicles (UAV) are ideal for multi-spectrum observation of large areas in different patterns (Kambouris 2018) and air-/ground- and surface/subsurface platforms (UAV/UGV/USV/UUV respectively) definitely for sampling, and possibly for distributing countermeasures. Highly integrated surveillance networks, cabled to similar ones used for public health, endowed with access to databases of medical interest are a first step in implementing awareness in those vast expanses.

The optimum setup of surveillance, despite the use of large-footprint technologies for surveillance and sampling, still needs to be dispersed in conducting the actual, technical part of an analysis (Kambouris et al. 2018, Kambouris et al. 2020). Although the development of IT and telecoms allows extreme fidelity in transducing images, sound and data (Herrera et al. 2014, Scherr et al. 2016), they can only assist in interpreting the actual lab results from afar; however, the results must be produced almost *in situ*, indicating a need for point of interest technologies and highly portable equipment (Priye et al. 2016). Even initial *in situ* processing of samples (with the widest of interpretations) is instrumental here, for it resolves the issue of the deterioration/decay of the sample and the degradation of the informational context, while also precluding carry-over contaminations and, of course, the overrun of centralized facilities that become high-demand and low-abundance resources in times of crises.

Bioeconomy: Opening the gates of ???????

The decisive turn towards a coupled concept of bioeconomy and circular economy seems to be a foregone conclusion in the early 2010s. Bioeconomy as understood today was defined in 2006 in a publication (Li et al. 2006) discussing China's prospects in an industry associated with biological applications. The earlier reports (1979 to 1992) used a more literal meaning of the term. In the ensuing years, the term had been established and culminated in a series of reports, insinuating a greater interest during the pandemic.

Bioeconomy is *not* necessarily cyclic; and cyclic economy need not be based on biological amenities (Venkatesh 2021). Any well-managed state would attempt a circular flow of goods and waste, whether within a bioeconomy or not; it is simply the logical thing to do. This scholarly digression notwithstanding, bioeconomy, especially if implemented from the start according to the principles of cyclic economy—something not very welcome in some corporate circles—would necessarily see a massive development of biotechnology and especially synthetic biology and bioengineering. The envisaged use of biological processes and practices will be unprecedented in all likelihood, both in volume and variety. Many of the enterprises will be outdoors, instead of roofed Centralized Processing Centers—CPCs (Polkinghorne 2018), to exploit space better and increase sustainability and affordability. The dispersed, as opposed to focal/concentrated, concept of economy implies such arrangements, while one of the primary objectives is to exploit currently non-productive 'wastelands' by applying the proper model of exploitation (as in low-enrichment surface ore deposits, by biomining) or by using technology to overcome limitations (as with the case of very low humidity/rainfall areas that are intended to be reclaimed for agriculture).

The aforementioned factors will increase the spatial footprint of what is now called 'agro sector' manifold and will also diversify it by introducing many new species—both microbial and others; while some of them would be wholly engineered or even xenobiotic (see Chapter 4), others would bear simpler upgrades to natural species. Among these are the genetically modified strains and the millennia-old practice of crossbreeds/hybrids, possibly with some methodological updates.

This implies novel populations with unknown qualities, not causing, but suffering, infectious diseases. As risky as the idea of the evolution of new or enhanced pathogens against humans and existentially related species (the Humanome) may sound (Kambouris et al. 2018b), it is comparatively a limited threat factor. The fact that a great proportion of life-sustaining world economic activity goes out of controlled areas/factories into the open, susceptible not only to weather and climate but also to infections, is a much riskier proposition. Under the current, unsustainable model, when a massive event occurs, it is usually focused locally or biologically; it impacts one species or a number of kin species (such as bovine). This allows for containment and also balancing by rerouting resources from other areas and sectors. This is not cost-effective and it is accompanied with great exploitation and corruption incidents and political leverage of the most unfair kind; however, it *does* allow for a degree of management of consequences and mitigation of the impact.

Given the nature of bioeconomy, many more sectors will be exposed to several other biorisks, leading to a rapid increase of the risk factor. On the other hand, the arrangements of a cyclic economy—a very cost-effective and efficient idea—mean that the derailment of one procedure would have a cascading effect on the *entire* network of activities, not limited to the downstream ones, regardless of any notion of transmissible pathogens; this is due to the cyclic arrangement. As a result, the *threat*, not the *risk* anymore, increases alarmingly fast. As the notions of sustainability, environmental protection and affordability are always present in financially-minded societies, there would be no alternative mechanism from which to transfer assets and resources exactly due to the magnitude of the disaster caused by the 'cyclic cascade'.

A cyclic economy needs relative precision in management, a prerequisite that in current economies is advisable but not necessary. The more integration there is, the more important precision becomes, and every divergence is amplified in terms of end effects. To put it plainly, a bioeconomy will cause systemic amplification of the impact of detrimental microbial interactions with the constituting elements, macrobiological or microbiological. In terms of biology, bioeconomy would offer much more advantageous conditions for the growth and transmission of existing potentially dangerous microorganisms; also, it is more likely to create much more favorable conditions for the evolution of even more aggressive and/ or fit microorganisms due to a wealth of genetic information in the form of ready sequences—to be integrated, tested and recombined—and a host-rich environment to allow the selection of evolved strains. The two biological effects may or may not combine with the systemic one mentioned before; if both biological effects occur and combine with the systemic projection, the omens seem unfavorable to the extreme.

The above lead to two prerogatives. First, in order to safeguard bioeconomy, the notion of biosecurity has to be greatly enhanced and diversified, rather than merely focusing on the production of edibles. It will be less resistant and robust in general terms as well as more prone to mistakes, which add up to increased vulnerability. Given the volume of the possibly affected entities, the biosecurity effort, implementable to the abovementioned risk factor, threat level and prospective impact, would be massive. It would even perhaps grow by orders of magnitude in terms resources compared to today's similar endeavors, and would comprise not only agrosecurity and industrial security, but also the biosecurity branch assigned to human subjects. The volume of surveillance, sampling, development of diagnostics and treatment, etc., would be much higher than even the expedited responses seen due to COVID-19. New technologies, approaches, infrastructure and synergies, along with command and control structures and communication needs, would be required. Agro sector workers would need security clearances on many occasions and training in 'good practices'—both of which are incompatible with the current standards of the workforce involved in such activities and which would be required for a much greater workforce than the one employed today.

Second, the agro sector will demand an investment in precision practices conceptually equivalent to, but methodologically distinct from, if not irrelevant to precision medicine and similar disciplines. This points towards the need for accurately applying biocides (pesticides, herbicides, etc.) and other (bio)chemical amenities, the accuracy pertaining to the type of molecule/regimen, dosage and host, all interrelated with the precise detection of the problematic spot and the thorough understanding of the etiology. As a result, the application would be strictly reactive and targeted and informed by precision diagnostics. This format would necessitate the replacement of many older generation wide-spectrum chemical compositions and establish the need for revisiting the rules for declaring a sample positive for an infectious agent. Else, the environmental footprint, the microbiomic deregulation and the financial cost of massively applied growth-enhancing and protective formulations (i.e., fertilizers and biocides of every kind) may heap severe deleterious effects in downstream stages of the cyclic economy, amplifying the ill effects without the presence of any threatening microbiomic agent.

Conclusion

Genomic homogeneity in most crops (King and Lively 2012, McDonald and Stukenbrock 2016) facilitates extreme propagation and effective dissemination of adapted pathogens, creating ever higher infectious loads. On the other end, a population group host of compromised immunity due to occasional (pregnancy, fatigue, seasonal or random diseases) or systematic (cancer, transplantation, HIV infection) events is bound to provide new hosts for cross-species hosting (Li et al. 2010, Kambouris et al. 2018b); these are susceptible despite being highly different than the pathogen's original source. Both the massive transportation of raw produce directly to marketing areas and the few immunodeficiency events in the most exposed rural populations create interfaces for new microbiota, especially fungi, to cross the host-species barrier, colonize and then adapt to human hosts, thus becoming opportunistic pathogens—a probabilistic event thus encouraged by the propagation of any single environmental contaminant. This mechanism might be responsible for the emerging and rare infections, especially those of fungal etiology.

Thus, given that most pathogens infiltrate into the human host from another source or reservoir (hostile interface), public health is extended to the agro sector and environment to survey tendencies and near-future infectious events. Molecular detection by medical protocols can be used for plant protection purposes, providing an early warning element for public health. Suitable protocols should be as generic as possible in order to be applied directly, or transferable, requiring the least adaptation possible. Some applicable techniques include New Generation Sequencing for dissecting the microbial populations by registering and identifying the constituting microbiota from plant, animal and soil samples; however, conventional, consensus-sequence PCR followed by RFLP is highly targetable and applicable in dispersed facilities for identifying pathogens at the species level (Kambouris et al. 2018a).

How disease is communicated in planetary distances and scale is demonstrated from the simple fact that the potato late blight of Ireland and the olive leaf blight in Apulia were brought about by pathogens native in America, which somehow found their way to the Old World. Whether these events were spontaneous (as was, most probably, the Mad Cow Disease in England in the 1990s) or not (as were the outbreaks of foot-and-mouth disease in sheep herds in NE Greece in the late 1990s) is conjectural. Still, it was a valid reason to dissuade high volumes of commerce for the sake of improved, and possibly more sustainable, local varieties instead of a diversified, concentrated and energy-intensive trade model, which ruthlessly exploits local shortages and based on massive transportation and fuel expenditure. In the long run, it was a mistake all along, but the agrosecurity aspect made it catastrophic. Contrary to some projections for human travel as a similarly risky proposal, the much lower volume, the massive investment in understanding human and microbiome interaction and integration, and the insurance sector make these events less possible, with the exception of immigration where no rules and no public health protocols are followed by the immigrants and the transporters/facilitators, making the biorisk transmission level similar to that for livestock, or even higher, given the strict rules of some countries in matters of imported foodstuff, and the hygiene and quality protocols.

The lower priority in terms of possible host populations, compared to human disease, makes the agro sector a perfect field for the application of current and latest technologies. Artificial intelligence may help in better assessing raw data returned from standard physical testing. One may even balance the given and irreversible relative shortage of real resources for surveying, testing and assessing the attributes of the agro sector by better exploiting the available physical primary data through different levels of processing filters.

The diseases in the agro sector spread much faster because surveillance, diagnostics and therapeutics therein receive much lower investments than the respective human (or even pet) sector(s). Additionally, the very dense growth conditions in intensive farming and breeding processes create a very friendly, host-rich environment for any communicable pathogen. The effect is further amplified since the cultivars and bloodlines are selected for profitability and not fitness, and are thus much less prone to sport efficient immune responses. This is one of the reasons for respective drug abuses, both in terms of quantity and pattern. A good example of the latter is the proactive administration of antibiotics to livestock in extremely dense growth formats, in mass-produced chicken for instance. It follows that Biosurveillance, meant to detect early and contain promptly, any such outbreak, faces additional challenges compared to its iterations concerned with human populations. Similarly, although occasionally isolation and quarantining is easier, massive decontamination and distribution of prophylactic and therapeutic amenities is vital, which allows a privileged niche for the use of innovative such approaches, exemplified by- without being restricted to- electromagnetic amenities (Chapter 8) and a wide spectrum of biologicals/biopharmaceuticals/biotherapeutics (Chapter 7), the latter applied in basic and occasionally advanced forms already (Manoussopoulos et al. 2019).

References

Adami, L. and Schiavon, M. (2021). From circular economy to circular ecology: A review on the solution of environmental problems through circular waste management approaches. Sustainability, 13(2): 925. doi: 10.3390/SU13020925.

Anderson, J.A. et al. (2019). Genetically engineered crops: Importance of diversified integrated pest management for agricultural sustainability. Frontiers in Bioengineering and Biotechnology, 24. doi: 10.3389/FBIOE.2019.00024/BIBTEX.

Ban, J. (2000). Agricultural Biological Warfare: An Overview, Office of Justice Programs. Available at: https://www.ojp.gov/ncjrs/virtual-library/abstracts/agricultural-biological-warfare-overview (Accessed: 23 August 2022).

Bawa, A.S. and Anilakumar, K.R. (2013). Genetically modified foods: safety, risks and public concerns-a review. Journal of Food Science and Technology, 50(6): 1035–1046. doi: 10.1007/S13197-012-0899-1.

Bötsch, M. (2004). SWISS AGRICULTURAL POLICY. Berne.

Claus, P. (2020). Author Reexamines Greek Famine During Years of Nazi Occupation, Greek Reporter. Available at: https://greekreporter.com/2020/10/21/author-reexamines-greek-famine-during-years-of-nazi-occupation/(Accessed: 23 August 2022).

Cockell, C.S. et al. (2020). Space station biomining experiment demonstrates rare earth element extraction in microgravity and Mars gravity. Nature Communications, 11(1): 1–11. doi: 10.1038/s41467-020-19276-w.

DeOtte, R.E. (2007). Agrosecurity for concentrated animal feeding operations (CAFOs): commentary on recent planning activities. Animal Health Research Reviews, 8(1): 89–103. doi: 10.1017/S1466252307001284.

Fraser, E.D.G. (2003). Social vulnerability and ecological fragility: Building bridges between social and natural sciences using the Irish Potato famine as a case study. Ecology and Society, 7(2): 9–18. doi: 10.5751/es-00534-070209.

Graziosi, A. (2004). The Soviet 1931–1933 Famines and the Ukrainian Holodomor: Is a new interpretation possible, and what would its consequences be? Harvard Ukrainian Studies, 27(1): 97–115.

Gyles, C. (2010). Agroterrorism. The Canadian Veterinary Journal = La Revue Veterinaire Canadienne, 51(4): 347–348. doi: 10.1081/e-eas2-120041359.

Herrera, S. et al. (2014). Field evaluation of an automated RDT reader and data management device for *Plasmodium falciparum/Plasmodium vivax* malaria in endemic areas of Colombia. Malaria Journal, 13(1). doi: 10.1186/1475-2875-13-87.

Janssen, D.B. and Stucki, G. (2020). Perspectives of genetically engineered microbes for groundwater bioremediation. Environmental Science: Processes and Impacts, 22(3): 487–499. doi: 10.1039/c9em00601j.

Kageyama, B. (2021). Why Winston Churchill Stopped Operation Vegetarian, History of Yesterday. Available at: https://historyofyesterday.com/why-winston-churchill-stopped-operation-vegetarian-e1c0a2176f04 (Accessed: 24 August 2022).

Kambouris, M.E. (2018). Mobile stand-off and stand-in surveillance against biowarfare and bioterrorism agents. pp. 241–55. *In*: Karampelas, P. and Bourlai, T. (eds.). Advanced Sciences and Technologies for Security Applications. Springer, doi: 10.1007/978-3-319-68533-5_12.

Kambouris, M.E. et al. (2018). Humanome versus microbiome: games of dominance and pan-biosurveillance in the Omics Universe. OMICS A Journal of Integrative Biology, 22(8): 528–538. doi: 10.1089/omi.2018.0096.

Kambouris, M.E. et al. (2018). Toward decentralized agrigenomic surveillance? A polymerase chain reaction-restriction fragment length polymorphism approach for adaptable and rapid detection of user-defined fungal pathogens in potato crops. OMICS A Journal of Integrative Biology, 22(4): 264–73. doi: 10.1089/omi.2018.0012.

Kambouris, M.E. et al. (2020). A focal point in GCBR and biosecurity. pp. 333–60. *In*: Kambouris, M.E. and Velegraki, A. (eds.). Microbiomics: Dimensions, Applications and Translational Implications of Human and Environmental Microbiome Research. ELSEVIER ACADEMIC PRESS.

Kambouris, M.E. et al. (2020). Point-of-need molecular processing of biosamples using portable instrumentation to reduce turnaround time. Biosafety and Health. Elsevier BV, 2(3): 177–82. doi: 10.1016/j.bsheal.2020.06.001.

Kambouris, M.E. and Velegraki, A. (2020). Myc(et)obiome: The big uncle in the family. pp. 29–51. *In*: Kambouris, M.E. and Velegraki, A. (eds.). Microbiomics: Dimensions, Applications, and Translational Implications of Human and Environmental Microbiome Research. 1st edn. London: Elsevier.

Kaur, T. (2019). Agro-Warfare: Attack on crops and livestock. CBW Magazine, 12(2).

King, K.C. and Lively, C.M. (2012). Does genetic diversity limit disease spread in natural host populations? Heredity, 109(4): 199–203. doi: 10.1038/hdy.2012.33.

Knowles, T. et al. (2005). Defining Law Enforcement's Role in Protecting American Agriculture from Agroterrorism. Washington, D.C.

Kramlich, D. (2014). Introduction to complementary, alternative, and traditional therapies. Critical care nurse, 34(6): 50–6; quiz 57. doi: 10.4037/ccn2014807.

Kurup, V.P. et al. (2000). Respiratory fungal allergy. Microbes and Infection, 2(9): 1101–1110. doi: 10.1016/S1286-4579(00)01264-8.

Lau, S.-E. et al. (2022). Microbiome engineering and plant biostimulants for sustainable crop improvement and mitigation of biotic and abiotic stresses. Discover Food, 2(1): 1–23. doi: 10.1007/S44187-022-00009-5.

Li, L. et al. (2010). Bat guano virome: predominance of dietary viruses from insects and plants plus novel mammalian viruses. Journal of Virology, 84(14): 6955–65. doi: 10.1128/JVI.00501-10.

Li, Q. et al. (2006). Biotechnology and bioeconomy in China. Biotechnology Journal, 1(11): 1205–1214. doi: 10.1002/BIOT.200600133.

Li, Z. et al. (2019). Pathogenic fungal infection in the lung. Frontiers in Immunology, 10: 1524. doi: 10.3389/FIMMU.2019.01524/XML/NLM.

Manoussopoulos, Y. et al. (2019). Effects of three strawberry entomopathogenic fungi on the prefeeding behavior of the Aphid *Myzus persicae*. Journal of Insect Behavior, 32(2): 99–108. doi: 10.1007/s10905-019-09709-w.

Marrero, J. et al. (2015). Recovery of nickel and cobalt from laterite tailings by reductive dissolution under aerobic conditions using acidithiobacillus species. Environmental Science and Technology. American Chemical Society, 49(11): 6674–6682. doi: 10.1021/ACS.EST.5B00944/SUPPL_FILE/ES5B00944_SI_001.PDF.

McDonald, B.A. and Stukenbrock, E.H. (2016). Rapid emergence of pathogens in agro-ecosystems: global threats to agricultural sustainability and food security. Philosophical transactions of the Royal Society of London. Series B, Biological sciences, 371(1709). doi: 10.1098/RSTB.2016.0026.

Monke, J. (2004). Agroterrorism: Threats and Preparedness. Washington, D.C.

Olsen, A. (2003). U.S. Moves Towards Biological Warfare in Colombia, PANNA. Available at: https://www.panna.org/legacy/panups/panup_20030124.dv.html (Accessed: 23 August 2022).

Owens, S. (2001). Salt of the earth. Genetic engineering may help to reclaim agricultural land lost due to salinisation. EMBO reports, 2(10): 877–879. doi: 10.1093/embo-reports/kve219.

Özdemir, V. (2018). The dark side of the moon: The internet of things, industry 4.0, and the quantified Planet. OMICS: A Journal of Integrative Biology, 22(10): 637–641. doi: 10.1089/omi.2018.0143.

Özdemir, V. (2021). From the Editor's Desk: Systems Science 2010–2020, and Post-COVID-19. Omics : a Journal of Integrative Biology. OMICS, 25(2): 73–75. doi: 10.1089/OMI.2021.0002.

Phippen, J. (2016). Kill Every Buffalo You Can! Every Buffalo Dead Is an Indian Gone'. The Atlantic. Available at: https://www.theatlantic.com/national/archive/2016/05/the-buffalo-killers/482349/ (Accessed: 23 August 2022).

Polkinghorne, R. (2018). From commodity, to customer, to consumer: The Australian beef industry evolution. Animal frontiers : The Review Magazine of Animal Agriculture, 8(3): 47–52. doi: 10.1093/af/vfy012.

Pravecek, T. et al. (2006). DoD Roles and Responsibilities. Maxwell AFB, Alabama.

Priye, A. et al. (2016). Lab-on-a-Drone: Toward pinpoint deployment of smartphone-enabled nucleic acid-based diagnostics for mobile health care. Analytical Chemistry. American Chemical Society, 88(9): 4651–4660. doi: 10.1021/acs.analchem.5b04153.

Pujawan, I.N. and Bah, A.U. (2021). Supply chains under COVID-19 disruptions: Literature review and research agenda. https://doi.org/10.1080/16258312.2021.1932568. Taylor & Francis, 23(1): 81–95. doi: 10.1080/16258312.2021.1932568.

Rogers, P. et al. (1999). Biological Warfare against Crops. Scientific American, 280(6): 70–5.

Rosie, G. (2001). UK planned to wipe out Germany with anthrax. The Glasgow Herald Sun, 14 October.

Ryan, L. (2018). Agro-warfare: The basics, SOFREP. Available at: https://sofrep.com/news/agro-warfare-basics/ (Accessed: 23 August 2022).

Satijn, H.M.C. and de Boks, P.A. (1988). Biorestoration, a technique for remedial action on industrial sites. Contaminated Soil '88. Springer, Dordrecht, pp. 745–753. doi: 10.1007/978-94-009-2807-7_120.

Scherr, T.F. et al. (2016). Mobile phone imaging and cloud-based analysis for standardized malaria detection and reporting. Scientific Reports. Nature Publishing Group, 6. doi: 10.1038/srep28645.

Seralini, G.E. (2020). Update on long-term toxicity of agricultural GMOs tolerant to roundup. Environmental Sciences Europe. Springer, 32(1): 1–7. doi: 10.1186/S12302-020-0296-8/METRICS.

Singh, L. et al. (2020). Eco-rejuvenation of degraded land by microbe assisted bamboo plantation. Industrial Crops and Products. Elsevier, 155: 112795. doi: 10.1016/J.INDCROP.2020.112795.

Steinhäuser, K.G. (2001). Environmental risks of chemicals and genetically modified organisms: A comparison. Environmental Science and Pollution Research. Springer Science and Business Media LLC, 8(3). doi: 10.1007/BF02987395.

Suman, J. et al. (2022). Microbiome as a key player in sustainable agriculture and human health. Frontiers in Soil Science. Frontiers, 2(2022): 12. doi: 10.3389/FSOIL.2022.821589.

Tenenbaum, D.J. (2008). Food vs. fuel: diversion of crops could cause more hunger. Environmental health perspectives. National Institute of Environmental Health Sciences, 116(6): A254. doi: 10.1289/EHP.116-A254.

Thomas, G. and De Tavernier, J. (2017). Farmer-suicide in India: debating the role of biotechnology. Life Sciences, Society and Policy. SpringerOpen, 13(1). doi: 10.1186/S40504-017-0052-Z.

Tooze, A. (2006). The Wages of Destruction. London: Allen Lane.

Unknown. (2017). Reforming agricultural subsidies to support biodiversity in Switzerland, OECD ENVIRONMENT POLICY PAPER. 8. Paris.

Unknown. (2022). SEAL History: Underwater Demolition Teams in the Korean War, National Navy UDT-SEAL Museum. Available at: https://www.navysealmuseum.org/naval-special-warfare/seal-history-underwater-demolition-teams-in-the-korean-war (Accessed: 23 August 2022).

Velegraki, A. and Zerva, L. (2020). Identifying microbiota: genomic, mass-spectrometric, and serodiagnostic approaches. pp. 77–94. *In*: Kambouris, M. and Velegraki, A. (eds.). Microbiomics: Dimensions, applications and translational implications of human and environmental microbiome research. ELSEVIER ACADEMIC PRESS.

Venkatesh, G. (2021). Circular Bio-economy—Paradigm for the future: Systematic review of scientific journal publications from 2015 to 2021. Circular Economy and Sustainability 2021 2:1. Springer, 2(1): 231–279. doi: 10.1007/S43615-021-00084-3.

Verma, N. and Sharma, R. (2017). Bioremediation of toxic heavy metals: A patent review. Recent Patents on Biotechnology, 11(3). doi: 10.2174/1872208311666170111111631.

Wankhede, P. and Wanjari, M. (2021). Health issues and impact of waste on municipal waste handlers: A review. Journal of Pharmaceutical Research International. Sciencedomain International, 33(46B), pp. 577–581. doi: 10.9734/JPRI/2021/V33I46B32979.

Woody, C. (2020). High-tech body armor of the future could come from spider butts, We Are The Mighty. Available at: https://www.wearethemighty.com/mighty-trending/body-armor-spider-silk/ (Accessed: 10 August 2022).

3

The Enemy in the Dish
Current and Projected Foodborne Biorisks and Liabilities

M. Kakagianni* and I. Giavasis*

Introduction

Food safety is a scientific discipline required for food security, which ensures that food will not harm the consumer's health at the point of consumption when prepared and/or eaten according to its intended use (Codex Alimentarius Commission 2020, Elmi 2004, Escanciano and Santos-Vijande 2014, International Organization for Standardization 2005, Jaffee et al. 2018). Given the recognized and microbiological hazards of food unsafe for human health, food safety has received increased international attention from farm to fork for all stakeholders worldwide (Bhat et al. 2021, Unnevehr 2015). *'Food safety equals behavior'* (Yiannas 2015), underlining the need to strengthen food safety culture and behavioral approaches to improve food safety performance. Rapid urbanization, intensification of animal breeding and crop farming, and globalization of food trade of raw materials as well as final products have resulted in a global interconnectedness and several changes in dietary habits, along with adaptations in food production, consumption and distribution patterns. These global changes have yielded not only a better coverage of nutritional needs of consumers, but also a wider and faster spread of food diseases among humans, thus posing new food safety challenges (Sankarankutty 2014). Nutrition and food safety are two sides of the same coin, inextricably linked to health (WHO 2021a). Food safety risks appear to be higher in general for foods with higher demand.

Department of Food Science and Nutrition, School of Agricultural Sciences, University of Thessaly, Karditsa, Greece.
* Co-corresponding authors: mkakagianni@uth.gr, ORCID iD: https://orcid.org/0000-0003-2278-8882; igiavasis@uth.gr, ORCID iD: https://orcid.org/0000-0001-9066-1627

The most traded foods—meat and fish products, as well as fruits and vegetables—are more frequently associated with food hazards and they also come from a wider range of countries now than they did a few decades ago. These factors pose a challenge to food safety authorities because of the increased risk associated with the lack of uniformity in food handling, manufacturing and transportation regulations across all the countries involved in the international food trade (Chammem et al. 2018). Despite increased efficiency and integration in food supply chains (te Brinke et al. 2022), food safety issues may arise as a result of increasing antimicrobial resistance, and human exposure to pesticides, antibiotics and other chemicals or pathogens contaminating agricultural products (e.g., crops, livestock, and fish) or drinking water (Aworh 2021, Mangla et al. 2021). Consequently, food safety is dependent on the somewhat predictable behavior of chemical and biological entities as well as the behavior of humans who perform more or less predictable activities in order to achieve a certain level of food safety as deemed acceptable by local and global standards. Thus, food safety is a socio-natural process (Busch 2004).

In the era of blockchain technology and traceability, a massive amount of digital data is generated in the agro-food industry, which could help in microbial risk evaluation and supervision, decision-making regarding the level of each threat, and ultimately the prevention of outbreaks (Kumarathunga 2020, Mirabelli and Solina 2020). Furthermore (Nayak and Waterson 2019), the food system is a complex socio-technical system that is intertwined with several other sectors, including water, energy, trade, agriculture, nutrition, and health, at various stages of food production, from initial processing to final home preparation and handling of the food product (Arora et al. 2018, Morse et al. 2018). Therefore, food safety issues should be managed not only at a national level (micro-level) but also at a global level (macro-level), due to globalization and market uncertainty and fluidity (Sazvar et al. 2018). Rapid and precise monitoring and detection of foodborne pathogens is required to ensure food safety throughout the production chain, prevent foodborne infections in humans and maintain hygiene standards for good health (Arora et al. 2018). Food safety and biosecurity are becoming increasingly important priorities of public health worldwide as the world's population grows and earth's resources dwindle. Despite recent technological advances, local policies, better public awareness and extensive investments in modern monitoring and control systems, foodborne diseases remain a widespread and growing public health concern in both developed and developing countries (Arora et al. 2018, Aworh 2021, Saravanan et al. 2021, WHO 2021a). Stringent legislation, supportive regulatory environmental policies, efficient food control systems and aligned standards must be established for the food supply chain to maintain high levels of food safety (Katsikouli et al. 2021, Zhang et al. 2018). In order to safeguard public health, regulators and risk assessment bodies must identify emerging food safety risks at an early stage (EFSA 2018). The circular economy now aims to control and improve global food security through sustainable production, as well as mitigate food safety crises through coordination and proper preparation of all involved stakeholders, primarily through the effective implementation of a comprehensive regulatory framework in the 'farm to fork' food chain (Chammem et al. 2018, Flynn et al. 2019, Gomez-Zavaglia et al. 2020, Tirado et al. 2010). However, global challenges such as climate change, urbanization and food (especially protein) shortage for the ever-expanding world population will continue to pose challenges for food safety in the future (Flynn et al. 2019). Thus, the main question is how to ensure food safety while increasing the productivity, complexity and interconnectivity of food production and supply chains. Keeping the food supply safe is an ongoing task that needs to adapt to the current state of food production and consumption. It is necessary to establish cooperation among food supply chain partners in order to improve quality assurance and reduce the cost of ensuring food safety (Smith and Fratamico 2018). In this context, 'One Health Initiative' has emerged in recent years, stating that we must begin at the farm level, with pathogen-controlled feed and healthy livestock, in a healthy environment, to ensure food safety (Kahn 2017). The concept of 'One Health' is the idea that human, animal, and environmental health are all interconnected. This approach engages multidisciplinary teams of academicians, producers, consumers, and government agencies that work together to achieve food security for the global population, preserve natural resources and improve health by safeguarding food safety and abiding to the nutritional requirements of a healthy diet (Sorbo et al. 2022).

This chapter discusses the impact of various factors that determine food safety nowadays—such as globalization, climate change, the complexity of the food supply chain, food fraud, pandemic crisis, and digital or other modern technologies of food protection. It also provides an overview of the potential tools available for examining and safeguarding food safety at European or even international levels.

Emerging food pathogens

Despite the ongoing progress towards safer food production, new biological, environmental and socio-economic challenges emerge at the surveillance, manufacturing and consumer levels. Outbreak investigations may reveal new pathogens, new food vectors and previously unknown gaps in the food safety framework (Nelluri and Thota 2018). Changes in the agro-food chain, social changes, and advancements in detection and reporting systems, combined with bacterial adaptation and evolution, may result in new and emerging zoonotic pathogens. For example, shigatoxigenic/enterohaemorrhagic *E. coli* (STEC/EHEC) and *Campylobacter* spp. in the meat chain; *Listeria monocytogenes* in vegetable, meat or milk products; *Cronobacter* spp. in infant milk formula; *Arcobacter* spp., *Yersinia enterocolitica* serobiotype O3/4, parasites such as *Cyclospora* on fruits; *Cryptosporidium* and *Giarda* in water; and Hepatitis E virus in pork and boar meat (Batzilla et al. 2011, Ramees et al. 2017). Recognizing current zoonotic pathogens and their potential for foodborne transmission is critical for detecting emerging foodborne pathogens. Also, as the analytical methods for the detection of biological hazards improve, new potential threats are revealed, such as emerging mycotoxins (enniatins, beauvericin, moniliformin, fusaproliferin, fusaric acid, culmorin, butenolide, sterigmatocystin, emodin, mycophenolic acid, alternariol, alternariol monomethyl ether, and tenuazonic acid) for which there are no regulatory limits of tolerance and thus no routine control and detection (Gruber-Dorninger et al. 2017).

Foodborne pathogens. Zoonotic diseases, which are transmitted to humans from animal hosts, have emerged as a result of a lack of food-safety standards monitoring and enforcement in food systems. In managed production systems and wildlife trade, improper animal storage, unsanitary conditions and poor handling of livestock products have been identified as channels for viral strain mutations and cross-species transmissions (Destoumieux-Garzón et al. 2018, Han et al. 2016, Hassell et al. 2017).

Despite numerous advancements in food safety measures and stricter inspection protocols, non-typhoidal *Salmonella* and *Campylobacter* continue to be the leading pathogens causing ever-increasing food safety concerns in the poultry (including fresh meat, minced meat, meat preparations and meat products) processing industry (EFSA 2019, Heredia and García 2018). Given some of the concerns raised about sampling and *Salmonella* recovery, relying solely on prevalence data to predict food safety appears to be a relatively inaccurate and potentially unreliable metric (O'Bryan et al. 2022). Not surprisingly, the prevalence of *Salmonella* in poultry products alone is not a good indicator of product safety, and a process risk model at the poultry processing plant level has been considered to be more likely to impact food safety (Oscar 2021). Several food safety scandals in the egg industry have occurred in recent years, causing consumer concerns, such as the *Salmonella* outbreak in the US in 2015 (Li et al. 2017, Whiley and Ross 2015). *Salmonella enterica* sub *enterica* serotype Hessarek, an uncommon serotype which can penetrate the eggshell, especially at room temperature (but less so under refrigeration), has recently emerged in foodborne salmonellosis as a result of consumption of contaminated eggs and egg products (Lin et al. 2021). The formation of biofilms and the development of stress tolerance, such as acid and heat tolerance in *Salmonella* as well as aerotolerance/oxygen tolerance in *Campylobacter*, are among the new food safety challenges (Thames and Theradiyil Sukumaran 2020). The use of antimicrobial agents in feed and foodborne diseases caused by these resistant bacteria in humans are well documented and have been linked to the growing resistance of foodborne zoonotic bacteria such as *Salmonella* spp. and *Campylobacter* spp. (Sorbo et al. 2022). *Salmonella* prevention requires controls that begin with poultry production at the farm and continue until the processed products reach the consumer's plate. In 2018, the WHO issued recommendations for *Salmonella* control that apply to the entire food chain (WHO 2018). Aside from food safety management programs based on prerequisite programs and HACCP covering the various stages of production, all food handlers must be trained and retrained on food safety on a regular basis, especially when dealing with ready-to-eat (RTE) foods in order to improve their knowledge of food handling and food poisoning and to sustain the industry (CIoF 2019, Ehuwa et al. 2021). These efforts are aimed at strengthening food safety standards to improve *Salmonella* surveillance efforts, educating consumers and training food handlers on best practices for preventing *Salmonella* and other foodborne diseases (WHO 2018). This means that well-trained food handlers with sufficient food safety knowledge can reduce the risk of food hazards (Yu et al. 2018). An example is the 2012 *E. coli* O157 outbreak in Canada, where the management's failure to provide adequate food safety training resulted in the absence of product recall protocols (Jespersen et al. 2017).

L. monocytogenes is still a major food safety risk and its elimination is a top priority in the EU. The unique physiological and ecological characteristics of this highly lethal pathogen widespread in soil, vegetables, animal feed and dairy and meat products, which can grow under refrigeration, while being relatively heat resistant to low temperature pasteurization, make it a real threat for the safety of low processed or ready-to-eat foods. For the latter a post-packaging treatment (thermal or non-thermal, High Hydrostatic Pressure for instance) could ensure food safety (Vidovic et al. 2022). Well-monitored sanitation of potentially infected surfaces and equipment (see also Chapters 5, 6 and 9) is critical for inhibiting the spread of this pathogen and implementing corrective measures; however, modern methods of quick detection of *L. monocytogenes* in foods or food facilities—where it can persist for long periods of time—are urgently needed (Ferreira et al. 2014). In fact, there is an obvious business opportunity for the development and commercialization of methods capable of *in situ* detection of *L. monocytogenes* quickly and reliably (Rodríguez-Herrera et al. 2021). Several optical, piezoelectric, cell-based and electrochemical biosensors for the early detection of *L. monocytogenes* in the food supply chain have been reviewed (Soni et al. 2018).

Bacillus cereus (*B. cereus*) is a novel emerging pathogen that has extensively contaminated animal feed and food chains, posing a significant economic loss to the food industry as well as a high risk to human health. This pathogen is a robust, omnipresent, heat-resistant spore former capable of forming biofilms; it is isolated from various environments (such as food and atmosphere) all year round, with no specific geographical distribution. It can cause serious food safety issues as it is difficult to ensure its absolute absence from food. Regulation focuses on *B. cereus* food safety limits (maximum tolerable limit) of 10^3 cfu/g in dairy products for the general public, 10^2 cfu/g in infant formula and 10^3 cfu/g in ready-to-eat meat and egg products. The amount of *B. cereus* spores in powdered infant formula and dried dietary foods is kept as low as possible throughout processing and thus high hygiene standards must be established throughout processing and distribution (Di pinto et al. 2013, Haque et al. 2021). Other members of this genus, such as *B. subtilis*, *B. licheniformis*, *B. pumilus*, *B. amyloliquifaciens*, *B. mojavensis*, *B. firmus*, *B. circulans*, *B. lentus*, *B. thuringiensis*, *B. megaterium*, *B. simplex*, *B. fusiformis*, *B. brevis* and *B. coagulans* have been deemed negligible and ignored in episodes of food poisoning; however, their existence and subsequent toxin outputs similar to emetic and enterotoxins have been increasingly documented as food safety concerns (Griffiths 2009, Logan 2012). Over one-third of probiotics in China's national survey between 2016 and 2018 contained antibiotic resistant strains, implying that probiotics found in commercial food items (meats and seafood) may be a means for transferring antibiotic resistance to food pathogens, posing a potential risk to public health (Fu et al. 2020). Therefore, it is vital to monitor the development of multi-drug resistance patterns in the *B. cereus* group in the food chain, and study its potential links to the sources of drug resistance. With the widespread and often unregulated use of probiotics in many countries (especially outside Europe), as well as their antimicrobial resistance profiles, stringent regulations are urgently required to reduce health risks associated with *B. cereus* and other pathogens (Haque et al. 2021).

Moreover, a growing concern for the global population is the presence of mycotoxins in foods of plant origin, as well as in dairy products. These potentially allergenic, hepatotoxic, inflammatory, immunotoxic or carcinogenic secondary metabolites of several fungi are very widespread and pose a health threat to both humans and animals (Gao et al. 2020, Vandenbroucke et al. 2011). Although approximately 500 mycotoxins have been identified from different fungi, health concerns are usually related to aflatoxins (AFs), ochratoxin A (OTA), deoxynivalenol (DON), fumonisins (FBs), zearalenone (ZEN), patulin (PAT), nivalenol (NIV) and citrinin (CTN) (Gao et al. 2020). Climate change exacerbates crop protection and food storage (see Chapter 5). For instance, there is evidence that water stress due to elevated temperatures can stimulate mycotoxin synthesis in some fungi (Magan et al. 2011). Furthermore, an increased prevalence of fungicide- or preservative-resistant fungal strains has been documented, resulting from the overuse of single-target fungicides and evolving market demands for longer shelf life of perishable food products (Davies et al. 2021). Interestingly, mycotoxins like deoxynivalenol, aflatoxins and ochratoxin A can also have a detrimental effect on the integrity of the intestinal barrier in both animals and humans and, thus, cause intestinal dysfunction or mycotoxicosis, or pave the way for intestinal inflammation by *Salmonella* or other pathogens within the gut microbiome (Gao et al. 2020, Vandenbroucke et al. 2011).

Food authenticity and food fraud

Food chain integrity encompasses microbial and chemical food safety, authenticity, fraud and quality throughout the food chain—from producers to consumers (Hoorfar et al. 2011). Food safety, food fraud and food defence incidents can result in food adulteration, posing public health risks. On the other hand, food authentication has become a major concern worldwide due to the globalization of food markets, in order to ensure food safety and avoid origin and quality fraud (Markiewicz-Keszycka et al. 2019). Spink and Moyer (2011) defined food fraud broadly as an illegal deception for economic gain; since then, the phenomenon, despite being an age-old problem, has been extensively reviewed and conceptualized. Food fraud vulnerability is defined by the Global Food Safety Initiative (GFSI 2017, 2018) as the "susceptibility or exposure to a food fraud risk, which is regarded as a gap or deficiency that could place consumer health at risk if not addressed." Food fraud is one of the components of the food risk continuum, which also includes food quality and safety concerns, along with food defense (Fritsche 2018, Spink et al. 2019a,b). Food fraud is the intentional or deliberate modification of food products and/or associated documentation for economic or financial gain, but the public's health is jeopardized (Manning and Soon 2019). The root cause(s) for food fraud are completely different from what is known about food safety. The driving force behind food adulteration is to maximize revenue by either using a cheap ingredient to (partially) substitute a more expensive one or by (partially) removing the higher valued component in the hope that the altered product goes undetected by the final user or consumer; watering of milk or skimming off cream are examples of such malpractices (Barnett et al. 2016, Ulberth 2020). However, if contamination occurs unintentionally, it is not a fraudulent act, but a food safety incident posing a public health risk and raising legal and/or quality concerns depending on the activities undertaken or the agent(s) used (Busta and Kennedy 2011, Manning and Soon 2019, Robson et al. 2021, Spink et al. 2017, Spink 2019).

Food fraud/adulteration and food authenticity are important aspects of food integrity, along with food standards, food assurance, food safety, food quality, food crime, food defense and food protection (Manning 2017, Wang et al. 2017). Food adulteration is considered more dangerous than traditional food safety threats in some cases as the potential adulterants are unconventional (e.g., the addition of melamine in infant formula to increase the apparent protein content of milk) and the impact is significant (e.g., melamine adulteration, also known as China's International Milk Crisis) (BBC 2010, Selamat and Iqbal 2016, Xin and Stone 2008). It was a tipping point that demonstrated how adulteration can have global ramifications, affecting consumers, businesses, industries and countries (Ellis et al. 2012). This scandal is not only about economic fraud but also about food safety. Food safety concerns arise when milk or milk products are substituted or adulterated with undeclared species (Hossain et al. 2021). The horsemeat scandal in the UK in 2012 is another example of fraudulent infiltration in the supply chain, rather than food safety *per se*. The substituted horsemeat was not detected quickly or even routinely in this case, for the UK beef industry relied on food safety strategies to trigger intervention (Spink et al. 2017). The scandal was only revealed through random DNA testing of products (Lawrence 2013), emphasizing the need for food suppliers to recognize and prioritize food fraud and food safety risks as distinct and important areas of concern (Spink and Moyer 2011, Spink et al. 2017, Tähkäpää et al. 2015). Another example is that the level of food safety in the Netherlands is high, but the opportunities for food fraud have also increased with fraudsters doing everything possible to avoid detection by the supervisory authority (NVWA 2018a). Furthermore, olive oil is always imported from Southern Europe, resulting in a longer supply chain and greater opportunity for fraud. The Netherlands' food policy prescribes a detailed food safety control system, but it does not specifically address food fraud (NVWA 2017, 2018b). Although most food fraud cases are motivated by financial gain, food fraud can also have direct and/or indirect consequences on food safety in many cases (Brooks et al. 2021). While food safety control can be well established in some developed countries, food authenticity for the purposes of food fraud necessitates greater cooperation as it involves cross-border transactions and the cooperation of several countries' law enforcement offices working against other financial crime and customs violations (Dutfield and Suthersanen 2022).

The EU Food Fraud Network, the UK Food Standards Agency (FSA-UK), the GFSI, the Safe Supply of Affordable Food Everywhere (SSAFE), the U.S. Pharmacopeia (USP), the U.S. Food and Drug Administration (FDA) and the Chinese National Center for Food Safety Risk Assessment (CFSA) are all important players in the fight against food fraud. Governments are holding competent food authorities accountable for safeguarding against all food risks and vulnerabilities, along with food safety and food authenticity or food fraud as a result of the impact on economies and consumer confidence, according to EU Regulation 2017/625. RASFF was established in the EU as a part of Regulation (EC) 178/2002 to aid in the control and safety of food and animal feed on the European market. The RASFF database contains both intentional food frauds, such as fraudulent documents or cases of adulteration, and unintentional frauds, such as improper, expired or missing documents (Fritsche 2018). Furthermore, the food industry is beginning to separate food fraud from food safety and food defence. The first step in this system is prevention, which is accomplished through HACCP and pre-requisite programs as the risks of food safety are well known. However, the matters of food fraud prevention and control (i.e., intentional acts committed for financial gain) fall beyond the scope of traditional HACCP-based food safety management systems as the adulterant in food frauds is often unknown (van Ruth et al. 2017). Said HACCP-based systems are not effective in detecting an infinite number of unknown adulterants (Moore et al. 2012, Robson et al. 2020). Counterfeit products, which are look-alikes of popular foods that are not produced with the same food safety assurances (Spink and Moyer 2011), pose a threat to the food industry and public health, for these products are unlikely to meet the required standards of hygiene or quality checks, significantly increasing the risks of a food safety outbreak (Moore et al. 2012). In contrast to food safety risk assessment which examines processes, a system to assess food fraud risk focuses on the factors involved as food products move along the supply chain and the environment in which this occurs (Ulberth 2020). However, the current risk analysis approach for food safety must be revised in order to provide evidence and guidance for developing policies to reduce food fraud incidents (Spink et al. 2019a,b). Several food safety management systems, which are widely used to ensure compliance with the EU food laws, have recognized the significance of food fraud as a risk factor and included food fraud vulnerability assessments and mitigation plans in their pre-requisite conditions for certification (Global Food Safety Initiative 2018). Indeed, there has been a push to incorporate risk assessments or food fraud vulnerability assessments into third-party industry food safety and quality standards (for example, Global Standard for food safety, version 8, BRC 2018a), mandating the food industry to identify weaknesses and/or criticalities within their processing facilities or supply chains. BRC Global Standard for Food Safety Issue 8 requires food manufacturers to conduct a documented vulnerability assessment on raw food materials to assess potential risks of adulteration or substitution (BRC Global Standards 2018a,b). However, the methodology of assessment is up to the manufacturers. PAS 96:2017 defines Campden Threat Assessment and Critical Control Point (TACCP) as the "systematic management of risk through the evaluation of threats, identification of vulnerabilities and implementation of controls of the entire production process." TACCP controls economic motivated adulteration (EMA) and malicious contamination, extortion, espionage, counterfeiting and cybercrime. It is concerned with identifying specific criminal and malicious threats to food safety (Swainson 2018) and is used in conjunction with Vulnerability Assessment and Critical Control Point (VACCP). The latter deals with the susceptibility of food fraud. Its scope includes the systematic prevention of potential food adulteration, intentional or unintentional, through the identification of vulnerable points in the supply chain (Global Food Safety Resource 2019). When it comes to fraud, FSSC 22000 (Food Safety System Certification) Version 4, HARPC (Hazard Analysis and Riskbased Preventive Controls) and TACCP (Threat Assessment Critical Control Points) appear to be essential within food industry standards. GFSI presented their strategy for incorporating food fraud into their Food Safety Management System in 2014. They shifted their focus from risks to vulnerabilities and defined the Food Safety Management Umbrella as three distinct pillars that must be addressed separately: HACCP (hazard/food safety), TACCP (threat/food defense) and VACCP (vulnerability/food fraud) (Kowalska 2018). Many countries make TACCP and

VACCP voluntary, whereas all food facilities in the US must establish and implement an adequate HARPC plan, mandating them to identify food safety and adulteration hazards, implement controls, design and implement corrective actions and verify the plan (Manning and Kowalska 2021). Food fraud vulnerability assessment (FFVA) tools differ from traditional purely food safety hazard analysis or risk assessment tools in that FFVA takes several socioeconomic factors into account. GFSIs as well as the WHO recognize FFVA as a critical requirement for an effective food fraud mitigation plan. FFVA is particularly useful for identifying flaws or weaknesses that allow for undesirable events to occur (Manning and Soon 2019, Spink et al. 2017). HorizonScan's original, a privatized subscription-based system that compiles alerts from governments around the world, including recalls, market withdrawals and other controls related to both food safety and food fraud, is one of the data sources available for food fraud vulnerability assessments (FERA 2018). Its primary goal is to detect emerging food safety threats before they become larger problems/risks in the food supply chain; it has also been expanded to include food integrity in general, including adulteration and food fraud (Food and Environment Research Agency (FERA) 2018, Manning and Soon 2019). The Food Protection and Defense Institute (FPDI) created the Food Protection and Defense Institute's World Factbook of Food; the World Factbook of Food contains information on the production, trade, seasonality, processing steps, supply chain structure, food safety concerns and past food fraud incidents for each product (FPDI 2017). The database, which is available on a subscription basis, was created to serve as a central reference database for food (DEFRA 2020).

While internal controls are critical, regulatory controls are required to enforce food safety regulations (FSA 2018). In this context, Article 19 of the EU food law for the prevention of food fraud (European Parliament & European Union Council 2019) requires food business operators to withdraw and recall food products when they believe they are not in compliance with the food safety requirements. In response to the European Parliament's request, the European Commission Directorate-General Health and Food Safety (DG SANTE) established a dedicated EU Food Fraud Network, installed a dedicated IT tool for food fraud related information exchange among Member States (Administrative Assistance and Cooperation System, AAC), and organized Coordinated Control Plans and dedicated training under the Better Training for Safer Food program (Ulberth 2020). Nowadays, it is widespread throughout the world, particularly in developing countries, though the full extent of adulteration is not conclusively known. This is primarily due to the fact that most incidents go unnoticed or unreported because they do not pose a food safety risk and consumers do not generally notice any quality issue associated with the adulterated food products as the adulterant components are usually very similar to the authentic product (Alamprese et al. 2013). In this context, traceability and authentication are essential components of the food safety and defense system, as well as fundamental components of the food supply chain. They are critical tools for assuring consumers' protection in terms of transparency, food safety and quality, allowing producers to become more aware of food authenticity, and connecting producers and consumers (Aung and Chang 2014, Fanelli et al. 2021). Food safety and quality authorities have requested an extended and updated list of analytical techniques for food authentication and assisting law enforcement (Dimitrakopoulou and Vantarakis 2021). Several studies have attempted to summarize various aspects of determining food authenticity, such as the country of origin, reactions to specific food fraud cases and the public attitude towards food safety as they relate to traceability (Bentivoglio et al. 2019). The use of chemometric models for authentication and provenance is regarded as a powerful tool for protecting geographically labeled rice and is especially useful for determining the origin of heavy metal contaminated rice and allowing government authorities to respond quickly to food safety risk events (Liu et al. 2019). Multiclass methods which analyze a large number of compounds in a single assay are becoming increasingly important in order to reduce the workload of the control laboratory workloads (Gavage et al. 2021, Steiner et al. 2021). Some authenticity testing systems, however, are ineffective when cases of fraud do not pose a significant risk to food safety (Brooks et al. 2021). High-Performance Liquid Chromatography (HPLC) is widely used for food authentication and is one of the most effective technologies for addressing food safety issues and ensuring that food is authentic in order to eliminate fraud (Selamat et al. 2021). The use of this technology is increasing, as is the number of available Ion Mobility Spectrometry (IMS)-based methods, particularly in the field of food safety and authentication. Despite the fact that IMS is an old technique, its application in the field of food safety and authenticity is yet to be thoroughly investigated. Furthermore, the fingerprinting approach has a lot of potential for food authentication (te Brinke et al. 2022). With the regulatory environment surrounding food safety and authenticity becoming more stringent, the importance of routine high-throughput control techniques is growing. The use of Next Generation Sequencing (NGS) has the ability to address multiple issues of authenticity and food safety simultaneously, providing exhaustive controls that may be especially important when dealing with new providers, ensuring consumer trust and protecting brand reputation (Haynes et al. 2019). Proteomics, lipidomics, metabolomics, metagenomics and transcriptomics are powerful tools for surveying food production, assessing food safety, authenticity and quality, detecting adulterations, allergens and toxins, and are involved in nutrigenomics research targeted at human well-being (Afzaal et al. 2022, Balkir et al. 2021, Josić et al. 2017). Metabolomics offers a broader range of analytical and detection options for food authentication, which may improve food quality and preserve food safety. The ongoing revolution in the metabolomics approach would make a significant contribution to the food industry's ability to maintain food safety and quality (Selamat et al. 2021). Digital polymerase chain reaction (dPCR) has also been shown to be very reliable and accurate in the control of food safety and adulteration. Techniques based on isothermal amplification have been shown to be highly sensitive and efficient in agro-food authentication and traceability (Fanelli et al. 2021). In short, the complex challenges of food safety and authentication necessitate data management systems capable of calculating variables and elements apart from the univariate model (Charlebois et al. 2021).

COVID-19 pandemic crisis and food safety

The COVID-19 pandemic has resulted in historical shifts in our society's norms and interactions. Although the WHO has stated that food is not a mode of transmission for COVID-19 (WHO 2020), many authorities including the US Food and Drug Administration Agency (FDA 2021) and the European Food Safety Authority (EFSA 2020) continue to collect data on the virus' potential persistence on food and the exact intermediate host for this virus. In this context, various food items stored at low temperatures (such as meat, poultry, and seafood) should be inspected to ensure food safety against SARS-CoV-2. As a result, public food safety concerns in the post-COVID-19 era are widespread, particularly in Chinese outdoor or local food markets, and expertise in tools addressing them is limited (Han et al. 2021, Yang 2020). The emergence of COVID-19 emphasizes the importance of designing, promoting and enforcing food-safety standards in local food systems as a global priority in order to protect against such unintentional biosecurity threats. As the COVID-19 hazard may be long-lasting, developing an accurate and fast detection method for SARS-CoV-2 in food surfaces and in the surrounding environment is the only way to ensure food safety. Nevertheless, preventive action necessitates the acknowledgement of the fact that food safety is a global public good (Henson and Traill 1993, Unnevehr 2007).

In the long term, the pandemic had a direct and significant impact on the entire food sector, primarily in four areas: bioactive compounds, food safety, food security, and sustainability (Galanakis 2020). Despite the fact that the measures required to ensure food safety, security and sustainability are converging more than ever before, it is critical to avoid hazardous and illegal food products reaching the market due to shortages, false claims, or other (economic for instance) reasons (Galanakis et al. 2021). The impact of COVID-19 on agricultural and food system output, as well as the main challenges during the post-COVID-19 recovery period, will revolve around food trading and markets, food safety and food practices. Prior to the current pandemic, food safety research tended to focus on food handling practices in industrial and commercial kitchens (Baş et al. 2007, Chapman et al. 2010, Harris et al. 2018, Jevšnik et al. 2008). Commercial restaurants that have survived the pandemic must remain resilient in order to continue profitable operation, while adhering to the food safety practices recommended by sanitary regulations (de Freitas and Stedefeldt 2020). The long-established good hygiene practices and food safety management systems have been reintroduced, revised, improved and supplemented and should be maintained in food service well into the post-pandemic period; such measures and practices include physical separation, installation of physical barriers, adequate ventilation, improved cleaning protocols, and providing personal hygiene training to food workers (ICMSF 2020). Implementing these food safety practices would reduce the likelihood of pathogens contaminating foods, thus preventing foodborne infections and easing the burden on the public health system (FAO 2020).

Control measures to limit the spread of COVID-19 may have aided in the prevention of food contamination in both domestic and public settings. In particular, the lockdown measures adopted in 2020 (such as stay-at-home orders, prohibition of private gatherings, closures and restrictions imposed on restaurants, pubs and public catering establishments, along with canteens in schools, universities, workplaces) may have significantly reduced the food poisoning typically associated with these settings (e.g., food contamination by norovirus, bacterial toxins and *Salmonella*) (CDC 2016). Also, travel-related foodborne outbreaks may have been reduced as a result of restrictions on international travel and mobility.

Certainly, the diversion of technical and human resources during the pandemic, accompanied with a lack of coordination with public health and food safety departments, hospitals and diagnostic laboratories, may have hampered the identification and investigation of foodborne outbreaks (EFSA and ECDC 2021). On the other hand, the level of consumer trust during the health crisis may influence their decision regarding the adoption of certain recommended food safety behaviors. Sanitation, personal hygiene equipment (masks, gloves, etc.) and other safety and hygiene measures (washing and sanitizing hands, temperature monitoring, etc.), as well as frequent cleaning of domestic kitchens and public settings (shops, restaurants, etc.), may have reduced food contamination and hence contributed to a general improvement in food safety at the consumer level. This has most likely contributed to a reduction in outbreaks in domestic settings, demonstrating the importance of promoting food safety and appropriate hygiene practices in home kitchens (e.g., washing hands, wearing gloves, cleaning surfaces, etc.). The COVID-19 pandemic caused a significant increase in handwashing practices. Although handwashing is an essential food safety behavior and discontinuing it may result in an increase in foodborne illnesses (CDC 2016), many consumers may not associate this practice with food safety. As a result of this behavior, they may reduce their handwashing frequency after the pandemic. For this reason, food safety educators should be aware of the increased risk perceptions during a health crisis in order to guide consumers towards adopting good food-handling behaviors and habits and continuing them even after the pandemic has ended and the risk perceptions decreased (Thomas and Feng 2021).

Furthermore, as a result of the COVID-19 pandemic, food quality, safety and security, along with consumer awareness, guide agro-food businesses towards innovative partnerships to improve product quality and safety (Saguy 2016), as well as safer no-touch initiatives, which is an important topic for the future (Memon et al. 2021, Wicaksono et al. 2021). As a consequence, businesses are increasingly implementing various food safety and quality assurance standards and systems, such as ISO and HACCP, in order to improve traceability and control of the food supply chain (Ling and Wahab 2020). In addition to implementing these food health checks, food companies should be vigilant about the potential food safety risks associated with COVID-19, as highlighted by WHO (2021a). To eliminate or reduce the risk of food being contaminated by the virus from food workers, hygiene measures should be reinforced and refresher training on food hygiene principles should be provided (WHO 2021b). The FDA (2021) recommends four basic steps for food safety: clean, separate, cook and chill. However, food safety is not the only goal. The most difficult challenge for the food industry is to protect food workers from contracting COVID-19, to prevent virus exposure or transmission and to improve food hygiene and sanitation practices (Ceniti et al. 2021).

The key to avoiding another pandemic is to integrate One-Health knowledge on zoonotic diseases with food safety measures throughout the food value chain. Reorienting policy priorities away from disease control and toward prevention will improve international coordination efforts towards pandemic preparedness. Food safety labels and education about the importance of safe food will increase the demand and, in turn, the willingness to pay, for food safety as a product attribute.

This will hasten the adoption of food safety measures throughout the supply chain. Investments made today in food safety would be extremely cost-effective in terms of reconstruction. Furthermore, the expected benefits of the food safety approach include reduction of risk of the emergencing diseases and prevention of global economic losses caused by pandemics. As a result, a long-term global approach to food safety is required to prevent future pandemics and food system disruptions (Aiyar and Pingali 2020). Despite international standards, the domestic food chains of countries have varying levels of food safety and risk. Owing to the differences in available technologies, plant and livestock host factors, food production traditions, cultural differences and topographical or climatic conditions, these risks differ (McAllister 2018). The recovery package's main challenge will be to close the policy-implementation gap, making food safety and hygiene practices the new standard from farm to fork (Han et al. 2021). The response to COVID-19 by all stakeholders, including governments, the agri-food industry, regulators and consumers, has the potential to change food safety, and fostering such demand is dependent partly on future research on food safety costs, performance evaluation and risk communication (Roy 2020).

References

Afzaal, M. et al. (2022). Proteomics as a promising biomarker in food authentication, quality and safety: A review. Food Science and Nutrition. https://doi.org/10.1002/fsn3.2842.

Aiyar, A. and Pingali, P. (2020). Pandemics and food systems-towards a proactive food safety approach to disease prevention & management. Food Security, 12(4): 749–756. https://doi.org/10.1007/s12571-020-01074-3.

Alamprese, C. et al. (2013). Detection of minced beef adulteration with turkey meat by UV–vis, NIR and MIR spectroscopy. LWT-Food Science and Technology, 53(1): 225–232. https://doi.org/10.1016/j.lwt.2013.01.027.

Arora, S. et al. (2018). Detecting food borne pathogens using electrochemical biosensors: An overview. International Journal of Chemical Studies, 6(1): 1031–1039.

Aung, M.M. and Chang, Y.S. (2014). Traceability in a food supply chain: Safety and quality perspectives. Food Control, 39: 172–184. https://doi.org/10.1016/j.foodcont.2013.11.007.

Aworh, O.C. (2021). Food safety issues in fresh produce supply chain with particular reference to sub-Saharan Africa. Food Control, 123: 107737. https://doi.org/10.1016/j.foodcont.2020.107737.

Balkir, P. et al. (2021). Foodomics: A new approach in food quality and safety. Trends in Food Science and Technology, 108: 49–57. https://doi.org/10.1016/j.tifs.2020.11.028.

Barnett, J. et al. (2016). Consumers' confidence, reflections and response strategies following the horsemeat incident. Food Control, 59: 721–730. https://doi.org/10.1016/j.foodcont.2015.06.021.

Baş, M. et al. (2007). Difficulties and barriers for the implementing of HACCP and food safety systems in food businesses in Turkey. Food Control, 18(2): 124–130. https://doi.org/10.1016/j.foodcont.2005.09.002.

Batzilla, J. et al. (2011). Yersinia enterocolitica palearctica serobiotype O: 3/4-a successful group of emerging zoonotic pathogens. BMC Genomics, 12(1): 1–11. https://doi.org/10.1186/1471-2164-12-348.

BBC. (2010). Timeline: China milk scandal. http://news.bbc.co.uk/2/hi/asia-pacific/7720404.stm. Accessed 03 June 2022.

Bentivoglio, D. et al. (2019). Quality and origin of mountain food products: The new European label as a strategy for sustainable development. Journal of Mountain Science, 16(2): 428–440. https://doi.org/10.1007/s11629-018-4962-x.

Bhat, S.A. et al. (2021). Agriculture-food supply chain management based on blockchain and IoT: A narrative on enterprise blockchain interoperability. Agriculture, 12(1): 40. https://doi.org/10.3390/agriculture12010040.

BRC Global Standards. (2018a). Food safety. Available at: https://www.brcglobalstandards.com/brc-global-standards/food-safety/, Accessed date: 21 June 2022.

BRC Global Standards. (2018b). BRC global standard food safety version 8 (August 2018). London: BRC Global Standards.

Brooks, C. et al. (2021). A review of food fraud and food authenticity across the food supply chain, with an examination of the impact of the COVID-19 pandemic and Brexit on food industry. Food Control, 130: 108171. https://doi.org/10.1016/j.foodcont.2021.108171.

Busch, L. (2004). Grades and standards in the social construction of safe food. *In*: Lien, M. and Nerlich , B. (eds.). The Politics of Food (1st ed., pp. 163–178). Oxford: BERG.

Busta, F.F.F. and Kennedy, S.P. (2011). Defending the safety of the global food system from intentional contamination in a changing market. pp. 119–135. *In*: Advances in Food Protection. Springer, Dordrecht. https://doi.org/10.1007/978-94-007-1100-6_7.

Canadian Institute of Food Safety (CIoF). Why Food Safety Training Is Important 2019. Available online: https://www.foodsafety.ca/blog/why-food-safetytraining-important (accessed on 16 June 2022).

CDC (Centers for Disease Control and Prevention). (2016). Hygiene fast facts. https://www.cdc. gov/healthywater/hygiene/fast_facts.html.

Ceniti, C. et al. (2021). Food safety concerns in "COVID-19 era". Microbiology Research, 12(1): 53–68. https://doi.org/10.3390/microbiolres12010006.

Chammem, N. et al. (2018). Food crises and food safety incidents in European Union, United States, and Maghreb Area: current risk communication strategies and new approaches. Journal of AOAC International, 101(4): 923–938. https://doi.org/10.5740/jaoacint.17-0446.

Chapman, B. et al. (2010). Assessment of food safety practices of food service food handlers (risk assessment data): testing a communication intervention (evaluation of tools). J Food Prot, 73(6): 1101–1107. https://doi.org/10.4315/0362-028X-73.6.1101.

Charlebois, S. et al. (2021). A review of Canadian and international food safety systems: Issues and recommendations for the future. Comprehensive Reviews in Food Science and Food Safety, 20(5): 5043–5066. https://doi.org/10.1111/1541-4337.12816.

Codex Alimentarius Commission. (2020). General Principles of Food Hygiene; FAO: Rome, Italy; WHO: Geneva, Switzerland.

Davies, C.R. et al. (2021). Evolving challenges and strategies for fungal control in the food supply chain. Fungal Biology Reviews, 36: 15–26. https://doi.org/10.1016/j.fbr.2021.01.003.

de Freitas, R.S.G. and Stedefeldt, E. (2020). COVID-19 pandemic underlines the need to build resilience in commercial restaurants' food safety. Food Research International, 136: 109472. https://doi.org/10.1016/j.foodres.2020.109472.

DEFRA, United Kingdom Department for Environment, Food and Rural Affairs. (2020). Food fraud mitigation. Food Authenticity Network. Retrieved June 23, 2022, from http://www.foodauthenticity.uk/food-fraud-mitigation-guides#g1.

Destoumieux-Garzón, D. et al. (2018). The one health concept: 10 years old and a long road ahead. Frontiers in Veterinary Science, 14. https://doi.org/10.3389/fvets.2018.00014.

Di Pinto, A. et al. 2013. Occurence of potentially enterotoxigenic *Bacillus cereus* in infant milk powder. European Food Research and Technology, (2): 275–279. https://doi.org/10.1007/s00217-013-1988-8.

Dimitrakopoulou, M.E. and Vantarakis, A. (2021). Does traceability lead to food authentication? A systematic review from a European perspective. Food Reviews International, pp. 1–23. https://doi.org/10.1080/87559129.2021.1923028.

Dutfield, G. and Suthersanen, U. (2022). Responding to the global food fraud crisis: What is the role of intellectual property and trade law? Queen Mary Stud Int Law, (378). https://ssrn.com/abstract=4028589.

EFSA Scientific Committee. (2018). Guidance on uncertainty analysis in scientific assessments. Efsa Journal, 16(1): e05123. https://doi.org/10.2903/j.efsa.2018.5123.

EFSA Panel on Biological Hazards (EFSA BIOHAZ Panel). (2019). Salmonella control in poultry flocks and its public health impact. EFSA Journal, 17(2): e05596. https://doi.org/10.2903/j.efsa.2019.5596.

Ehuwa, O. et al. (2021). Salmonella, food safety and food handling practices. Foods, 10(5): 907. https://doi.org/10.3390/foods10050907.

Ellis, D.I. et al. (2012). Fingerprinting food: current technologies for the detection of food adulteration and contamination. Chemical Society Reviews, 41(17): 5706–5727.10.1039/C2CS35138B.

Elmi, M. (2004). Food safety: current situation, unaddressed issues and the emerging priorities. EMHJ-East Mediterranean Health Journal, 10(6): 794–800. https://apps.who.int/iris/handle/10665/119481.

Escanciano, C. and Santos-Vijande, M.L. (2014). Reasons and constraints to implementing an ISO 22000 food safety management system: Evidence from Spain. Food Control, 40: 50–57. https://doi.org/10.1016/j.foodcont.2013.11.032.

European Food Safety Authority, EFSA. (2020). Coronaviruses: No evidence that food is a source or transmission route. https://www.efsa.europa.eu/en/news/coronavirus-no-evidence-food-source-or-transmission-route/. (Accessed 24 June 2022).

European Food Safety Authority, & European Centre for Disease Prevention and Control. (2021). The European Union one health 2020 zoonoses report. EFSA Journal, 19(12): e06971. https://doi.org/10.2903/j.efsa.2021.6971.

European Parliament, & European Union Council. (2019). Regulation (EC) No 178/2002 of the European Parliament and of the Council of 28 January 2002 laying down the general principles and requirements of food law, establishing the European Food Safety Authority and laying down procedures in matters of food safety. Official Journal of the European Union 02002R0178-EN-26.07.2019-007.001.

Fanelli, V. et al. (2021). Molecular approaches to agri-food traceability and authentication: An updated review. Foods, 10(07): 1644. https://doi.org/10.3390/foods10071644.

FAO. (2020). Food safety in the time of COVID-19. https://doi.org/10.4060/ca8623en.

Flynn, K. et al. (2019). An introduction to current food safety needs. Trends in Food Science and Technology, 84: 1–3. https://doi.org/10.1016/j.tifs.2018.09.012.

FDA. (2021). Best practices for retail food stores, restaurants, and food pick-up/delivery services during the COVID-19. Available online: https://www.fda.gov/food/food-safety-during-emergencies/best-practices-retail-food-stores-restaurants-and-foodpick-updelivery-services-during-covid-19#employeehealth (accessed on 15 July 2022).

FPDI. Food Protection and Defense Institute. 2017. https://facts.foodprotection.io/about.

Ferreira, V. et al. (2014). Listeria monocytogenes persistence in food-associated environments: Epidemiology, strain characteristics, and implications for public health. Journal of Food Protection, 77(1): 150–170. https://doi.org/10.4315/0362-028X.JFP-13-150.

Food and Environment Research Agency (FERA). (2018). HorizonScan global food Integrity and risks system. Retrieved 23 June, 2022 https://www.fera.co.uk/media/wysiwyg/HorizonScan_Leaflet.pdf.

Fritsch, L. et al. (2019). Insights from genome-wide approaches to identify variants associated to phenotypes at pan-genome scale: Application to *L. monocytogenes*' ability to grow in cold conditions. International Journal of Food Microbiology, 291: 181–188. https://doi.org/10.1016/j.ijfoodmicro.2018.11.028.

Fritsche, J. (2018). Recent developments and digital perspectives in food safety and authenticity. Food Chemistry, 66(29): 7562–7567. https://doi.org/10.1021/acs.jafc.8b00843.

FSA. (2018). Managing food safety. Available at: https://www.food.gov.uk/businessguidance/managing-food-safety, Accessed date: 21 June 2022.

Fu, S. et al. (2020). National safety survey of animal-use commercial probiotics and their spillover effects from farm to humans: an emerging threat to public health. Clinical Infectious Diseases, 70(11): 2386–2395. https://doi.org/10.1093/cid/ciz642.

Galanakis, C.M. (2020). The food systems in the era of the coronavirus (COVID-19) pandemic crisis. Foods, 9(4): 523. https://doi.org/10.3390/foods9040523.

Galanakis, C.M. et al. (2021). Innovations and technology disruptions in the food sector within the COVID-19 pandemic and post-lockdown era. Trends in Food Science and Technology, 110: 193–200. https://doi.org/10.1016/j.tifs.2021.02.002.

Gao, Y. et al. (2020). The compromised intestinal barrier induced by mycotoxins. Toxins, 12(10): 619. https://doi.org/10.3390/toxins12100619.

Gavage, M. et al. (2021). Suitability of high-resolution mass spectrometry for routine analysis of small molecules in food, feed and water for safety and authenticity purposes: A review. Foods, 10(3): 601. https://doi.org/10.3390/foods10030601.

GFSI. GFSI benchmarking requirements version 7.2. 2017. https://www.mygfsi.com/certification/ benchmarking/gfsi-guidance-document.html. Accessed 21 June 2022.

Global Food Safety Initiative (GFSI). (2018). Tackling food fraud through food safety management systems. https://www.mygfsi.com/files/Technical_Documents/201805-foodfraud-technical-document-final.pdf (accessed 22 June 2022).

Global Food Safety Resource. (2019). TACCP and VACCP: What's the difference? Available at: https://globalfoodsafetyresource.com/taccp-and-vaccp-what-is-the-difference/Accessed date: 21 June 2022.

Gomez-Zavaglia, A. et al. (2020). Mitigation of emerging implications of climate change on food production systems. International Food Research Journal, 134: 109256. https://doi.org/10.1016/j.foodres.2020.109256.

Griffiths, M.W. (2009). *Bacillus cereus* and Other *Bacillus* spp. In Pathogens and Toxins in foods: Challenges and Interventions, 1–19. https://doi.org/10.1128/9781555815936.ch1.

Gruber-Dorninger, C. et al. (2017). Emerging mycotoxins: Beyond traditionally determined food contaminants. Journal of Agricultural and Food Chemistry, 65(33): 7052–7070. https://doi.org/10.1021/acs.jafc.6b03413.

Han, B.A. et al. (2016). Global patterns of zoonotic disease in mammals. Trends in Parasitology, 32(7): 565–577. https://doi.org/10.1016/j.pt.2016.04.007.

Han, S. et al. (2021). COVID-19 pandemic crisis and food safety: Implications and inactivation strategies. Trends in Food Science and Technology, 109: 25–36. https://doi.org/10.1016/j.tifs.2021.01.004.

Haque, M.A. et al. (2021). Pathogenicity of feed-borne *Bacillus cereus* and its implication on food safety. Agrobiological Records, 3: 1–16. https://doi.org/10.47278/journal.abr/2020.015.

Harris, K.J. et al. (2018). Foodborne illness outbreaks in restaurants and patrons' propensity to return. International Journal of Contemporary Hospitality Management, 30(3): 1273–1292. https://doi.org/10.1108/IJCHM-12-2016-0672.

Hassell, J.M. et al. (2017). Urbanization and disease emergence: dynamics at the wildlife–livestock–human interface. Trends in Ecology and Evolution, 32(1): 55–67. https://doi.org/10.1016/j.tree.2016.09.012.

Haynes, E. et al. (2019). The future of NGS (Next Generation Sequencing) analysis in testing food authenticity. Food Control, 101: 134–143. https://doi.org/10.1016/j.foodcont.2019.02.010.

Henson, S. and Traill, B. (1993). The demand for food safety: Market imperfections and the role of government. Food Policy, 18(2): 152–162. https://doi.org/10.1016/0306-9192(93)90023-5.

Heredia, N. and García, S. (2018). Animals as sources of food-borne pathogens: A review. Animal Nutrition, 4(3): 250–255. https://doi.org/10.1016/j.aninu.2018.04.006.

Hoorfar, J. et al. (eds.). (2011). Food chain integrity: A holistic approach to food traceability, safety, quality and authenticity. Elsevier.

Hossain, A. et al. (2021). Detection of species adulteration in meat products and Mozzarella-type cheeses using duplex PCR of mitochondrial cyt b gene: A food safety concern in Bangladesh. Food Chemistry: Molecular Sciences, 2: 100017. https://doi.org/10.1016/j.fochms.2021.100017.

ICMSF. (2020). ICMSF opinion on SARS-Cov-2 and its relationship to food safety. https://www.icmsf.org/wp-content/uploads/2020/09/ICMSF2020-Letterhead-COVID-19-opinion-final-03-Sept-2020.BF_.pdf.

International Organization for Standardization. (2005). Food safety management systems—Requirements for any organization in the food chain. Accessed 28 June 2022. Available at: https://www.iso.org/obp/ui#iso:std:iso:22000:ed-1:vl:en.

Jaffee, S. et al. (2018). The safe food imperative: Accelerating progress in low-and middle-income countries. World Bank Publications.

Jespersen, L. et al. (2017). Development and validation of a scale to capture social desirability in food safety culture. Food Control, 82: 42–47. https://doi.org/10.1016/j.foodcont.2017.06.010.

Jevšnik, M. et al. (2008). Food safety knowledge and practices among food handlers in Slovenia. Food Control, 19(12): 1107–1118. https://doi.org/10.1016/j.foodcont.2007.11.010.

Josić, D. et al. (2017). Use of foodomics for control of food processing and assessing of food safety. Advances in Food and Nutrition Research, 81: 187–229. https://doi.org/10.1016/bs.afnr.2016.12.001.

Kahn, L.H. (2017). Perspective: The one-health way. Nature, 543(7647): S47–S47. https://doi.org/10.1038/543S47a.

Katsikouli, P. et al. (2021). On the benefits and challenges of blockchains for managing food supply chains. Journal of the Science of Food and Agriculture, 101(6): 2175–2181. https://doi.org/10.1002/jsfa.10883.

Kowalska, A. (2018). The study of the intersection between food fraud/adulteration and authenticity. Acta Universitatis Agriculturae et Silviculturae Mendelianae Brunensis, 66(5): 1275–1286. https://doi.org/10.11118/actaun201866051275.

Kumarathunga, M. (2020, April). Improving farmers' participation in agri supply chains with blockchain and smart contracts. In 2020 Seventh International Conference on Software Defined Systems (SDS) (pp. 139–144). IEEE. 10.1109/SDS49854.2020.9143913.

Lawrence, F. (2013). Horsemeat scandal: The essential guide. The guardian: 15, 02–13. www.theguardian.com/uk/2013/feb/15/horsemeat-scandal-the-essential-guide (accessed 27 July 2022).

Li, T. et al. (2017). Consumer preferences before and after a food safety scare: An experimental analysis of the 2010 egg recall. Food Policy, 66: 25–34. https://doi.org/10.1016/j.foodpol.2016.11.008.

Lin, Q. et al. (2021). Salmonella Hessarek: An emerging food borne pathogen and its role in egg safety. Food Control, 125: 107996. https://doi.org/10.1016/j.foodcont.2021.107996.

Ling, E.K. and Wahab, S.N. (2020). Integrity of food supply chain: going beyond food safety and food quality. International Journal of Productivity and Quality Management, 29(2): 216–232.

Liu, Z. et al. (2019). Assuring food safety and traceability of polished rice from different production regions in China and Southeast Asia using chemometric models. Food Control, 99: 1–10. https://doi.org/10.1016/j.foodcont.2018.12.011.

Logan, N.A. (2012). Bacillus and relatives in foodborne illness. Journal of Applied Microbiology, 112(3): 417–429. https://doi.org/10.1111/j.1365-2672.2011.05204.x.

Magan, N. et al. (2011). Possible climate-change effects on mycotoxin contamination of food crops pre-and postharvest. Plant Pathology, 60(1): 150–163. https://doi.org/10.1111/j.1365-3059.2010.02412.x.

Mangla, S.K. et al. (2021). A framework to assess the challenges to food safety initiatives in an emerging economy. Journal of Cleaner Production, 284: 124709. https://doi.org/10.1016/j.jclepro.2020.124709.

Manning, L. (2017). Food integrity. Br Food J, 119(1): 2–6. http://doi.org/10.1108/BFJ-09-2016-0446.

Manning, L. and Kowalska, A. (2021). Considering fraud vulnerability associated with credence-based products such as organic food. Foods, 10(8): 1879. https://doi.org/10.3390/foods10081879.

Manning, L. and Soon, J.M. (2019). Food fraud vulnerability assessment: Reliable data sources and effective assessment approaches. Trends in Food Science and Technology, 91: 159–168. https://doi.org/10.1016/j.tifs.2019.07.007.

Markiewicz-Keszycka, M. et al. (2019). Laser-induced breakdown spectroscopy for food authentication. Current Opinion in Food Science, 28: 96–103. https://doi.org/10.1016/j.cofs.2019.10.002.

McAllister, S.R. (2018). Implementation of food safety regulations in food service establishments (Doctoral dissertation, Walden University).

Memon, S.U.R. et al. (2021). Investigation of COVID-19 impact on the food and beverages industry: China and India perspective. Foods, 10(5): 1069. https://doi.org/10.3390/foods10051069.

Mirabelli, G. and Solina, V. (2020). Blockchain and agricultural supply chains traceability: Research trends and future challenges. Procedia Manufacturing, 414–421. https://doi.org/10.1016/j.promfg.2020.02.054.

Moore, J.C. et al. (2012). Development and application of a database of food ingredient fraud and economically motivated adulteration from 1980 to 2010. Journal of Food Science, 77(4): R118–R126. https://doi.org/10.1111/j.1750-3841.2012.02657.x.

Morse, T.D. et al. (2018). Achieving an integrated approach to food safety and hygiene—Meeting the sustainable development goals in sub-saharan Africa. Sustainability, 10(7): 2394. https://doi.org/10.3390/su10072394.

Nayak, R. and Waterson, P. (2019). Review Global food safety as a complex adaptive system: Key concepts and future prospects. Trends in Food Science and Technology, 91: 409–425. https://doi.org/10.1016/j.tifs.2019.07.040.

Nelluri, K.D. and Thota, N.S. (2018). Challenges in emerging food-borne diseases. In Food safety and preservation (pp. 231–268). Academic Press. https://doi.org/10.1016/B978-0-12-814956-0.00009-3

NVWA. (2017). Multi annual national control plan (MANCP). https://english.nvwa.nl/about-us/multi-annual-national-control-plan-mancp Accessed 21 June 2022.

NVWA. (2018a). Food safety statement. https://english.nvwa.nl/binaries/nvwa-en/documents/consumers/food/safety/documents/food-safety-statement/food-safetystatement.pdf. Accessed 21 June 2022.

NVWA. (2018b). Dutch food safety is high, but opportunities for food fraud increase. https://english.nvwa.nl/news/news/2018/07/02/dutch-food-safety-is-high-butopportunities-for-food-fraud-increase. Accessed 21 June 2022.

O'Bryan, C.A. et al. (2022). Public health impact of *Salmonella* spp. on raw poultry: Current concepts and future prospects in the United States. Food Control, 132: 108539. https://doi.org/10.1016/j.foodcont.2021.108539.

Oscar, T. (2021). Salmonella prevalence alone is not a good indicator of poultry food safety. Risk Analysis, 41(1): 110–130. https://doi.org/10.1111/risa.13563.

PAS 96. (2017). Guide to protecting and defending food and drink from deliberate attack. Available at: https://www.food.gov.uk/sites/default/files/pas962017.pdf, Accessed date: 21 June 2022.

Ramees, T.P. et al. (2017). Arcobacter: An emerging food-borne zoonotic pathogen, its public health concerns and advances in diagnosis and control–a comprehensive review. Veterinary Quarterly, 37(1): 136–161. https://doi.org/10.1080/01652176.2017.1323355.

Robson, K. et al. (2020). A 20-year analysis of reported food fraud in the global beef supply chain. Food Control, 116: 107310. https://doi.org/10.1016/j.foodcont.2020.107310.

Robson, K. et al. (2021). A comprehensive review of food fraud terminologies and food fraud mitigation guides. Food Control, 120: 107516. https://doi.org/10.1016/j.foodcont.2020.107516.

Rodríguez-Herrera, J. et al. (2021). Methodological approaches for monitoring five major food safety hazards affecting food production in the Galicia–Northern Portugal Euroregion. Foods, 11(1): 84. https://doi.org/10.3390/foods11010084.

Roy, D. (2020). World food safety day 2020: COVID-19 offers an opportunity for India's food systems to deliver on safety and health. https://www.ifpri.org/blog/world-food-safety-day-2020-covid-19-offers-opportunity-indias-food-systems-deliver-safet y-and/. (Accessed 24 June 2022).

Saguy, I.S. (2016). Challenges and opportunities in food engineering: Modeling, virtualization, open innovation and social responsibility. Journal of Food Engineering, 176: 2–8. https://doi.org/10.1016/j.jfoodeng.2015.07.012.

Sankarankutty, K.M. (2014). Biosensors and their applications for ensuring food safety. Global Journal of Pathology and Microbiology, 2(1): 15–21.

Saravanan, A. et al. (2021). Methods of detection of food-borne pathogens: A review. Environmental Chemistry Letters, 19(1): 189–207. https://doi.org/10.1007/s10311-020-01072-z.

Sazvar, Z. et al. (2018). A sustainable supply chain for organic, conventional agro-food products: The role of demand substitution, climate change and public health. Journal of Cleaner Production, 194: 564–583. https://doi.org/10.1016/j.jclepro.2018.04.118.

Selamat, J. and Iqbal, S.Z. (eds.). (2016). Food safety: Basic concepts, recent issues, and future challenges. Springer. 10.1007/978-3-319-39253-0.

Selamat, J. et al. (2021). Application of the metabolomics approach in food authentication. Molecules, 26(24): 7565. https://doi.org/10.3390/molecules26247565.

Smith, J.L. and Fratamico, P.M. (2018). Emerging and re-emerging foodborne pathogens. Foodborne Pathogens and Disease, 15(12): 737–757. https://doi.org/10.1089/fpd.2018.2493.

Soni, D.K. et al. (2018). Biosensor for the detection of Listeria monocytogenes: emerging trends. Critical Reviews in Microbiology, 44(5): 590–608. https://doi.org/10.1080/1040841X.2018.1473331.

Sorbo, A. et al. (2022). Food safety assessment: Overview of metrological issues and regulatory aspects in the European Union. Separations, 9(2): 53. https://doi.org/10.3390/separations9020053.

Spink, J. and Moyer, D.C. (2011). Defining the public health threat of food fraud. Journal of Food Science, 76(9): R157–R163. https://doi.org/10.1111/j.1750-3841.2011.02417.x.

Spink, J. et al. (2017). Food fraud prevention shifts the food risk focus to vulnerability. Trends in Food Science and Technology, 62: 215–220. https://doi.org/10.1016/j.tifs.2017.02.012.

Spink, J. et al. (2019a). Global perspectives on food fraud: results from a WHO survey of members of the International Food Safety Authorities Network (INFOSAN). NPJ Science of Food, 3(1): 1–5. https://doi.org/10.1038/s41538-019-0044-x.

Spink, J. et al. (2019b). The application of public policy theory to the emerging food fraud risk: Next steps. Trends in Food Science and Technology, 85: 116–128. https://doi.org/10.1016/j.tifs.2019.01.002.

Spink, J.W. (2019). The current state of food fraud prevention: Overview and requirements to address 'How to Start?' and 'How Much is Enough?' Current Opinion in Food Science, 27: 130–138. https://doi.org/10.1016/j.cofs.2019.06.001.

Steiner, D. et al. (2021). Challenges and future directions in LC-MS-based multiclass method development for the quantification of food contaminants. Analytical and Bioanalytical Chemistry, 413(1): 25–34. https://doi.org/10.1007/s00216-020-03015-7.

Swainson, M. (2018). Swainson's handbook of technical and quality management for the food manufacturing sector. Woodhead Publishing.

Tähkäpää, S. et al. (2015). Patterns of food frauds and adulterations reported in the EU rapid alert system for food and feed and in Finland. Food Control, 47: 175–184. https://doi.org/10.1016/j.foodcont.2014.07.007.

te Brinke, E. et al. (2022). Insights of ion mobility spectrometry and its application on food safety and authenticity: A review. Analytica Chimica Acta, 340039. https://doi.org/10.1016/j.aca.2022.340039.

Thames, H.T. and Theradiyil Sukumaran, A. (2020). A review of Salmonella and Campylobacter in broiler meat: Emerging challenges and food safety measures. Foods, 9(6): 776. https://doi.org/10.3390/foods9060776.

Thomas, M.S. and Feng, Y. (2021). Consumer risk perception and trusted sources of food safety information during the COVID-19 pandemic. Food Control, 130: 108279. https://doi.org/10.1016/j.foodcont.2021.108279.

Tirado, M. et al. (2010). Climate change and food safety: A review. Food Res Int, 43(7): 1745–1765. https://doi.org/10.1016/j.foodres.2010.07.003.

Ulberth, F. (2020). Tools to combat food fraud–a gap analysis. Food Chemistry, 330: 127044. https://doi.org/10.1016/j.foodchem.2020.127044.

Unnevehr, L.J. (2007). Food safety as a global public good. Agricultural Economics, 37: 149–158. https://doi.org/10.1111/j.1574-0862.2007.00241.x.

Unnevehr, L. (2015). Food safety in developing countries: Moving beyond exports. Global Food Security, 4: 24–29. https://doi.org/10.1016/j.gfs.2014.12.001.

Vandenbroucke, V. et al. (2011). The mycotoxin deoxynivalenol potentiates intestinal inflammation by *Salmonella typhimurium* in porcine ileal loops. PloS one, 6(8): 23871. https://doi.org/10.1371/journal.pone.0023871.

van Ruth, S.M. et al. (2017). Food fraud vulnerability and its key factors. Trends in Food Science and Technology, 67: 70–75. https://doi.org/10.1016/j.tifs.2017.06.017.

Vidovic, S. et al. (2022). Lifestyle of *Listeria monocytogenes* and food safety: Emerging listericidal technologies in the food industry. Critical Reviews in Food Science and Nutrition, pp. 1–19. https://doi.org/10.1080/10408398.2022.2119205.

Wang, C.S. et al. (2017). Food integrity: a market-based solution. British Food Journal. https://doi.org/10.1108/BFJ-04-2016-0144.

Whiley, H. and Ross, K. (2015). Salmonella and eggs: From production to plate. International Journal of Environmental Research and Public Health, 12(3): 2543–2556. https://doi.org/10.3390/ijerph120302543.

Wicaksono, T. et al. (2021). Prioritizing business quality improvement of fresh agri-food SMEs through open innovation to survive the pandemic: A QFD-based model. Journal of Open Innovation: Technology, Market, and Complexity, 7(2): 156. https://doi.org/10.3390/joitmc7020156.

World Health Organization, WHO. Salmonella (non-typhoidal). (2018). Available online: https://www.who.int/news-room/fact-sheets/detail/Salmonella-(non-typhoidal) (accessed on 16 June 2022).

World Health Organization, WHO. (2020). COVID-19 and food safety: Guidance for food businesses. http://www.who.int/publications-detail/covid-19-and-food-safety-guidance-for-food-businesses. (Accessed 24 June 2022).

World Health Organization, WHO. (2021a). Draft WHO global strategy for food safety 2022–2030, towards stronger food safety systems and global cooperation, Department of Nutrition and Food Safety Prepared by WHO Secretariat. https://www.who.int/publications/m/item/draft-who-global-strategy-for-food-safety-2022-2030.

World Health Organization, WHO. (2021b). World Health Organization COVID-19 and Food Safety: Guidance for food Businesses: Interim Guidance. Available online: https://www.who.int/publications/i/item/covid-19-and-food-safety-guidance-for-food-businesses (accessed on 15 July 2022).

Xin, H. and Stone, R. (2008). Chinese probe unmasks high-tech adulteration with melamine. Science, 322(5906): 1310–1311. 10.1126/science.322.5906.1310.

Yang, X. (2020). Potential consequences of COVID-19 for sustainable meat consumption: The role of food safety concerns and responsibility attributions. British Food Journal. https://doi.org/10.1108/BFJ-04-2020-0332.

Yiannas, F. (2015). Food Safety= Behavior. New York: Springer Science Business Media, 10: 978–1. Doi: 10.1007/978-1-4939-2489-9.

Yu, H. et al. (2018). Implementation of behavior-based training can improve food service employees' handwashing frequencies, duration, and effectiveness. Cornell Hospitality Quaterly, 59(1): 70–77. https://doi.org/10.1177/1938965517704370.

Zhang, Z. et al. (2018). Transformation of China's food safety standard setting systeme-Review of 50 years of change, opportunities and challenges ahead. Food Control, 93: 106–111. https://doi.org/10.1016/j.foodcont.2018.05.047.

4

Beyond the Biosphere

M.E. Kambouris

Introduction

The establishment of a microbiote in a physically or functionally distinct environment, different from the original, may result in creating and occupying an entirely different niche. If its spontaneous adaptation is successful, the migration may be very aggressive; within the associated possible outcomes lies an increased pathogenicity over a range of hosts, which may very well cause extinction-level events, for the immune systems adapt rather slowly. Although there is enough residual flexibility in immune responses, especially but not exclusively innate, to tackle unknown contacts (Yokoyama and Colonna 2008, Obeng et al. 2021), more elaborate solutions need considerable depth of time; adequate immune response against parasites of metazoic pedigree is yet to occur (Davidson 1985).

Non-spontaneous, evolutionary adaptation (Obeng et al. 2021) may lead to the deletion of the immigrational event by the inbound agent conforming completely in some preexisting niche, or to a slower evolutionary adaptation of the microbiote; the key to the latter is its ability to endure and survive, perhaps at the level of mere sustenance, by not arousing adverse responses in the new habitat (Foster et al. 2017)—herein, the immune system of a host is but one among such responses. Other microbiota may well discourage later additions in the microbiome by secreting antimicrobial or other indirectly adverse agents like pH modifiers.

If alien microbiota appear, the most probable course of action would be spontaneous adaptation. The very nature of their novelty would rather preclude the ability to co-exist and co-evolve. They would be either incapable of adapting to the new environment or, on the contrary, uniquely fit. This duality of extremes has a

University of Patras, School of Health Sciences, Department of Pharmacy, Patras, Greece & The Golden Helix Foundation, London, United Kingdom.
Email: mekambouris@yahoo.com, ORCID iD: https://orcid.org/0000-0002-3205-4797

more sinister result: the possibility of inadaptability means low risk and, thus, low priority in respective bioresilience and R&D budget allocation, while the threat level remains extremely high, suggesting a GCBR-level event (Palmer et al. 2017).

The whole idea of Xenobiology rests upon the core of the alienation principle (Budisa et al. 2020), if seen from an evolutionary or even a creationist perspective. From the lens of actuality, it was all about pedigrees that could not interact genetically (although it is used for biochemical incompatibility as well in certain cases), given that biochemical incompatibility means no infection potential, at least of septic nature (a toxic effect remains possible if not highly probable) and limited predatory relationships, if any. The initial idea was that extraterrestrial life, usually denoted by 'exo-' or 'astro-' prefixes (Budisha et al. 2020), evolved in completely different environments, possibly on planets with different spectral type sun-stars which would loosely abide by the principles of life but were based on different, non-carbon biochemistries (Schulze-Makuch and Irwin 2006). Whether these lifeforms would have evolved along the lines similar to the Natural History of Earth is a valid query. If so, lifeforms similar to the ones observed at-planet (an expanded notion of the expression 'at-home') could be expected, as suggested by the Sci-Fi lore for decades.

There is of course the distinct possibility that alien life, even if fulfilling the prerogatives set for recognizing an entity as alive in earth, would be very different in form and function. This would further suggest difficulties in detecting, recognizing, studying and categorizing it, while a more ominous query arises: if there are forms of life undetectable due to their form and environmental signature, it would be conceivable to have some of those within the earthly biosphere already, while we have not been able to identify or apperceive them (shadow biosphere).

In essence, and as our horizons widen, the issue of alien lifeforms develops in various different axes (Box 4.1):

(i) Lifeforms similar to the types known to us, in terms of form and function, but developed beyond the biosphere independently and able to interact with our own or possibly intermingle: The second term suggests possibilities of exchange of genetic information and *in extremis* procreation of mixed pedigrees.

(ii) As in (i) but not *developed independently*, rather *evolved independently*: This suggests a common ancestry followed by some isolation event, and increases the interaction and intermingling potentials much higher.

(iii) Lifeforms similar to the terrestrial lifeforms in terms of function (possibly even in form, but this is not a prerequisite), but of other, carbon-based biochemistries: In these cases, the potential for interaction is high, but for intermingling is rather low.

(iv) Lifeforms similar to the terrestrial lifeforms in terms of form but of different biochemistries, originating in similar or vastly dissimilar environmental conditions.

> **Box 4.1. Different categories of alien life**
>
> - *Earth-like* life throughout the universe, originating through an extra-terrestrial creation event (McKay 2010) and followed by some kind of interspace dissemination, or through multiple similar creation events in different systems/planets, again followed by interspace transportation/communication. The realm of astrobiology *par excellence.*
> - Lifeforms totally different than the known ones (Schulze-Makuch and Irwin 2006), unidentified and/or unrecognized exactly due to unfamiliarity, but adapted to the geoenvironment and existing at certain locations in it or at its fringes; the object of Shadow Biosphere and the realm of astrobiology.
> - *Earth-like* life on-planet but alienated from common forms as it was developed and evolved beyond the biosphere, in enclaves formed by isolation events (Schulze-Makuch et al. 2017). This category could be the object of astrobiology, exobiology (in a more expansive interpretation) and xenobiology as well.
> - The forms of alien life developed independently out of the confines of the planet and with no functional resemblance in biochemistry to the biosphere analogues, while possibly developing similar morphologies, has been the initial focus of exobiology when the space exploration was initiated. It can be argued that following the Soviets, the term '*cosmobiology*' should be introduced to contain the whole of exo- and astrobiology along with the study of the Shadow Biosphere (which may in itself have analogues in space).
> - The purely synthetic/engineered lifeforms, made to present minimal or no compatibility with the living organisms as we know them today, are the core realm of synthetic xenobiology (Acevedo-Rocha and Budisa 2016, Völler and Budisa 2017, Schmidt et al. 2018, Budisa et al. 2020).

(v) Lifeforms significantly dissimilar from the recognized forms (irrespective of the similarity or dissimilarity of their native environment to the earth's biosphere) and thus somewhat cryptic, at least until they develop intelligence *and* propensity to communicate with dissimilar intelligences: Artificial Intelligence turning auto-cybernetic (Aguilar et al. 2014), and crystals (Schulman and Winfree 2008) are two popular examples, brought up simply to demonstrate the dynamics.

The other aspect is the expected horizon for alien lifeforms. The main idea for using the term 'alien' is beyond the biosphere, but this is much less straightforward than expected. It has spatial as well as temporal and functional considerations (not merely spatial, as is widely understood).

(I) The first and easy location of alien life would be out of the confines of the planet and thus clearly out of the biosphere. This, of course, changes with space travel and the resulting knowledge and understanding that occur in increments: other planets within the solar system, other planets beyond the solar system (termed 'exoplanets' and thus the name of the discipline being 'exobiology', at least initially), different iterations from other planetary systems or star systems, and ultimately other galaxies (Figure 4.1).

(II) The other location would be within the confines of the earth but beyond the biosphere, in enclaves formed by isolational events which would either restart an evolutionary process or guide the earthly evolution towards different pathways and results.

(III) Shadow Biosphere refers to totally different lifeforms within the boundaries of the planet (Figure 4.2), but which adapted to the geoenvironment, possibly even to the environment of the biosphere, but not yet identified as lifeforms due to the nature and intensity of the respective signatures (Cleland and Copley 2005, Cleland 2007).

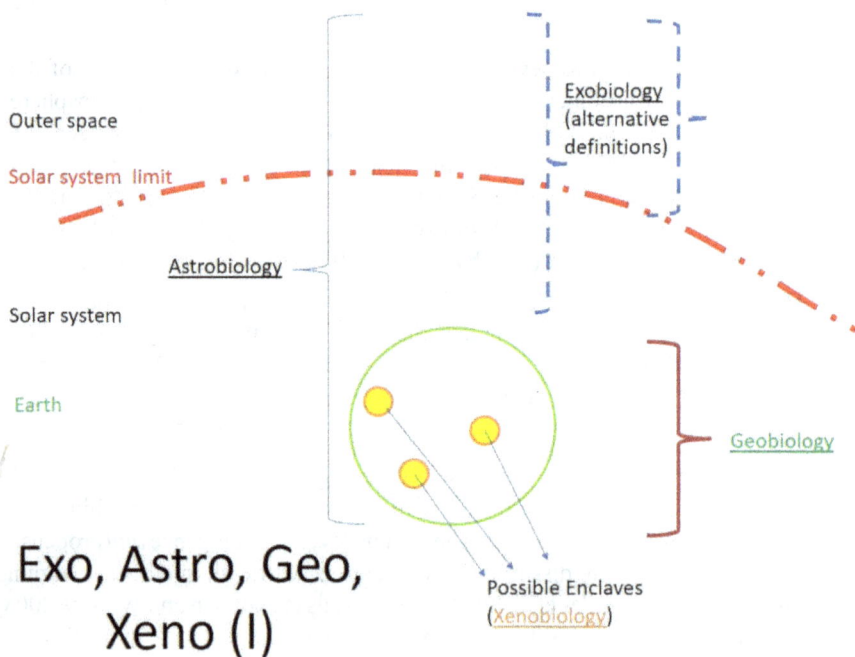

Figure 4.1. The spatial differentiation among Astrobiology, Exobiology and Geobiology and Xenobiology.

Exo, Astro, Geo, Xeno (II)

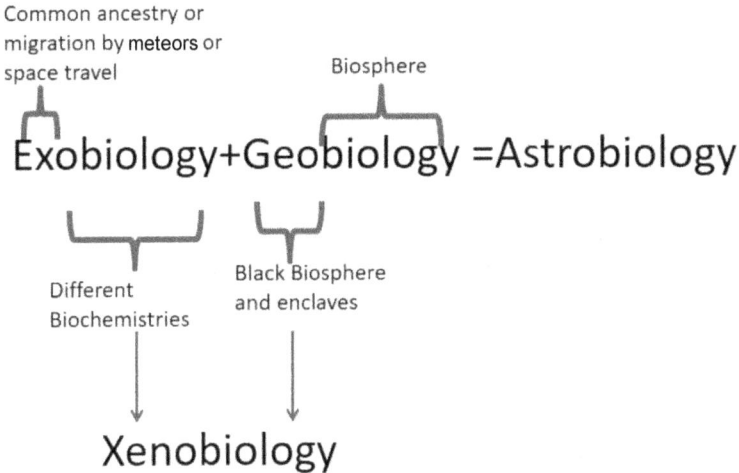

Common ancestry or
migration by **meteors** or
space travel

Biosphere

Exobiology+Geobiology =Astrobiology

Different
Biochemistries

Black Biosphere
and enclaves

Xenobiology

Figure 4.2. The semantic relation among Astrobiology, Exobiology and Geobiology and Xenobiology.

Definitions

The official NASA page refers to exobiology as the original name of the faculty concerned with extra-terrestrial life, now known as 'astrobiology' (NASA n.d. a). This implies that the two terms are virtually synonymous. There are, though, attempts to differentiate them (Unknown n.d.a) and the notion goes that Exobiology is named after the search and probability of life in Exoplanets (which orphans the planets and other celestial bodies within the solar system, like the Martians) while Astrobiology is more inclusive and includes Earth as well (Figure 4.1). This is a tad debatable: there is nothing in the word 'astrobiology' referring to the Earth; biology is about life as we know it, that is, on earth and perhaps on earthen appendices and ecosystems (like spacecrafts and spaceships or colonies). Thus, any such notion of the term 'astrobiology' is by definition redundant, especially once the term 'geobiology' came into use (NASA n.d.b), although obviously as a subset (hyponym) of 'astrobiology' (Figures 4.1 & 4.2).

Moreover, except for the case of space vessels, life is rather expected to develop on some planet and definitely not on a star proper; thus, astrobiology should actually imply the equivalent of exobiology: life on other planets orbiting stars other than the Sun but with a focus on being attached to solar systems and thus excluding rogue planets (NASA n.d.c).

These two terms focus on life beyond the physical reach of the biosphere of the earth, but in an explicit outward orientation, meaning space. Of the two, only astrobiology directly implies such restraints as a factor of semantics and terminology. Exobiology may refer to more inclusive areas of study and interest: first of all, other celestial bodies of the solar system, and then earthly locations severed from the actual biosphere if not from other earthen constants (such as the atmosphere and/or the hydrosphere). The 'exo-' prefix (Greek for 'out') can and should have been used more liberally and by itself, and not as a graft from the entity of exoplanets. Given the privileged status of classical studies in the 50's, actually the decade of infancy of the space exploration, one would expect that this was the intended meaning and use. A meaning that was much more attuned to the-then actual capabilities, as the exoplanets were definitely beyond NASA's reach, and it still remains doubtful whether at that time any of them had been properly located and identified. It would also fit well with the NASA-mandated explorations on earth, allegedly for extreme-environment research, but possibly for alien indigenous life signs, and of course the current iteration of Earth Sciences in NASA research interests (NASA n.d.d). One should not forget that the American Space Program pushed the concept of stars ('Astronaut'). On the contrary, the Soviets used the more inclusive term 'Cosmonaut', which was based on the less defined concept of *cosmos* (Greek for 'the world') and thus suggested 'beyond the earth', rather than the sometimes unrealistic fixation with other stars and star systems.

The missing, interpretive link may be the dynamic factor. Exobiology does study (prospectively) life that developed and evolved on other planets (Figure 4.1); astrobiology may have included Earth as a possibly non-originating part of life. The latter may have been actually produced as such in different locations in space and traveling, or being transported or transplanted in celestial bodies (Figure 4.2), the Earth included (McKay 2010). It is a temporally retrospective look within the universe for a single or possibly multiple migration events of a single pedigree and the different evolutionary paths taken by the isolations created by space barriers among the different incubation/receiver loci. Thus, astrobiology actually engages in the current and historic study of *earth-like* life throughout the Universe, which means an inherently high potential of intermingling and interacting, *along with* concerns regarding colonization through space—intentional (by space travel and colonies) or spontaneous (by lifeforms aboard meteors or other celestial trekking objects, including contaminants in spaceships). This version, which is not directly declared but subtly implied in open NASA sources assigns the study of entirely different lifeforms, such as the ones of non-carbon biochemistry (as understood in Sci-Fi lore), in the realm of exobiology, which is not a hyponym but another entity altogether, with a partial overlap with astrobiology. Additionally, if location stops being the defining issue and different lifeforms are included in the search horizon *on Earth*, meaning the shadow biosphere (Cleland and Copley 2005), astrobiology is still current; it would produce a competent bridge for associating different lifeforms from different celestial bodies, regardless of sequential or independent emergence.

The other key word is *Xenobiology* (Unknown n.d.b). The prefix xeno- means *foreigner* or *alien* in Greek and is regularly used to denote a complete lack of commonness or relatedness. For instance, in 'xenobiotic substances in the food chain', it refers to the basically unwarranted takeover of synthetic substances that cannot be produced or metabolized by the affected organism, including but not being limited to residues of plasticware and insecticides/pesticides, especially organophosphates (Croom 2012). The term is wide enough to encompass all cases of alien life, but, and this is a key component, also non-spontaneous forms; thus, it now includes the concept of synthetic biology for designing, developing and producing lifeforms of different iterations of functional genomics. This iteration may be minimal, confined to the genetic code, or much more elaborate, using slightly or entirely different metabolites. 'Slightly' implies different molecules of the same category as the mainstream biochemistry, for instance some additional *existing* nucleobases or amino acids which are not included in the current genetic codes (emphasis on plural). The use of entirely different monomers, as synthetic nucleobases, or other categories of macromolecules is reserved for the 'entirely different' category mentioned above.

Synthetic biology excluded, the original meaning of Xenobiology *sensu stricto* affiliates it rather to the exobiology spectrum of research, implying different lifeforms. The 'how different' is a valid query and a matter of definition: the extraterrestrial location of the same genetic code and biochemistry mechanisms in organisms bearing no resemblance and no functional or morphological relationship with the terrestrial ones, may qualify for xenobiological research. Or maybe not.

The security dimension of Aliens

Once space invasions are left out of the picture and the security spectrum is confined to the notion of infection and disease, or even parasitism, microbiome reshuffle and colonization, the basic attributes come into clear focus: the organisms presenting a direct biological threat (not an indirect threat through disruption) must bear a minimum commonality with the indigenous microbiome so as to effect exchanges, synergies or antagonisms and associations in general.

To present a threat, the novel microorganism—synthetic, extraterrestrial, stellar or from some forgotten cave in the bowels of the planet or from the ocean—must interfere and interact with the established biosphere. The lowest order of interaction is the abiotic environment—temperature, chemical environment, pressure, oxidative or reductive character of the atmosphere, compatibility with the residual forms and intensity of radiation (solar, radioactivity and cosmic rays included) and, very importantly, with the plentiful elements and molecules found in the biosphere (mainly in its abiotic part). The compatibility with water is something obvious, but Silicon and different minerals may be just as important, at least for non-carbon biochemistries that may be the cradle of life in planets with very different gravitational and atmospheric conditions.

A novel organism may use enzymes and evolutionary characteristics that are not recognizable patterns for the immune system of the probable hosts. The latter are defined by the presence of substances of interest as sources of energy or matter (carbon, nitrogen or ready-made macromolecules-actually nutrients) in their metabolome. Being able to parasitize and being unknown to the immune system is expected mainly to characterize xenobiota from secluded, isolated ecosystems that have digressed in evolutionary terms, as well as from space niches where life, as we know it, may have been transplanted or evolved *de novo*. If some niches of the current biosphere are permissive to such microbiota, they may proliferate and disperse uncontrollably, and any moiety proving antimicrobial activity against them would be a stroke of luck or, considering immunoglobulin-based mechanisms, the result of the conformational competence and adjustability of the epitope-paratope recognition system. An example of benign such organisms, are the prokaryotes using arsenic instead of phosphorus in their nucleic acids (Wolfe-Simon et al. 2011).

The said category may cause genomic/genetic pollution, passing codes that may provide entirely new attributes to existing microbiota. These attributes may be identical or similar to the ones the sequences in question were coding in their source organisms. But they also may not. This is a highly intriguing prospect: a random sequence may enter and become incorporated in a receiver genome. There, it might acquire a genetic meaning completely novel, due to its interpretation by the translational mechanism of the receiver genome and organism. This interpretation would depend on the receiver's genetic code and translational mechanism, especially regarding the open reading frame(s) and the identity of the Start and the Stop codons. But this may not be the case sometimes and the xenobiote may be genetically incompatible with the SBM (standard biosphere microbiota). This implies that genetic analysis, as we know it, may be inapplicable; even if applicable, it may detect the xenobiote but might not reveal much about its physiology for diagnostic testing or designing antimicrobial moieties, chemical or other. A long and laborious approach of massively testing material and energy regimens would be required to identify the liabilities and target moieties, along with developmental dynamics, from hypobiotic and polymorphic patterns to resistance factors, toxin production and nutrient uptake dynamics and kinetics. It must be stressed that, in certain cases, an obvious difference may be less than an absolute barrier. For example, it is conceivable that the genetic code of the As-genomed prokaryota may be read and is essentially similar to the standard versions, corrected for evolutionary level, *despite* the major difference in the backbone, with Arsenic instead of Phosphorus. But if the bases are the same, the code may be similar and also readable by standard PCR approaches edited for the different chemistry and interactions with the As-containing backbone. Even if the polymerases cannot work due exactly to the change in the backbone, hybridization-based approaches may be viable and allow a xenogenomic mapping. Same or similar principles may apply to proteome and metabolome research, and from there to structural studies and functional *in silico* simulations and prognosis.

Highly compatible xenobiota (Level 1 and 0, see Box 4.2) may cause immediate diseases in different taxa of the standard biosphere and kick-start evolutionary lines and traits, especially if they partake in genome exchange procedures or are amenable to the available ones (mainly transformation, transduction, transposition and conjugation). These xenobiota present the widest reaching risk factors, for they may cause evolutionary events and/or themselves become the objects of such events by receiving catabolism or resistance genes and initiating interactions differing in means (the kinds of biomolecules involved) or events (the procedures enacted by the biomolecules), for instance.

Nonetheless, they are biomolecules in the strict sense of the term and their physicochemical liabilities targeted by many antimicrobial interventions (including

Box 4.2. Xenobiota compatibility score

0 (Zero). Full compatibility. Identical biochemistry and genetics, with similar genetic code, standard translational machinery, use of identical primary macromolecules and possible lateral gene transfer. New species evolved under mid-term isolation or in standard speciation processes; extent of variability in the horizon of the known examples—within the Biosphere.

1. **High compatibility**

Genetic code similar or reproducible but not identical; elements are missing but the main sequence can be copied, amplified or transcribed and thus create genetic pollution, although the translation is different in the receiver organisms. The physiology has similar but different basic mechanisms, which are susceptible to similar stimuli and conditions, although the specter of susceptibility could be wildly varying. Highly evolved and specific antimicrobial amenities, such as antibiotics and antibody-defined responses and interventions (natural or technological) are not applicable deterministically, but some residual utility may be identified on a case-by-case basis perhaps in a stochastic fashion. More generic approaches, targeting specifically (or not) less well-defined entities and functions, may be moderately drastic in a case-by-case context. This context refers to groups wildly dissimilar; the common ground may be as narrow as any taxon or as wide as a given biosphere. This level of compatibility is expected from exoworlds and synthetic evolutionary lines, suggesting the study of exobiology, astrobiology and xenobiology.

2. **Medium compatibility**

The operative idea of synthetic xenobiology is that it introduces a vastly different genetic code, possibly but not necessarily intended to disallow any crosstalk with the existing one, either in translation or in interpretation. This status of incompatibility could also be a spontaneous, creationist event outside the premises of synthetic xenobiology, birthing a similar but different biochemistry. Except a genetic code based on different building blocks, including but not limited to a different code (different, incompatible bases of the nucleotides), differences may have been introduced in different levels of the physiology. For example, different isomers of biomolecules being introduced into the metabolome and considerably or even slightly different chemical groups (as in amino acids and nucleotides) having been preferentially included in the coding and engineering blueprints of lifeforms. On the other hand, material and procedural similarity allows thriving in subsets of the current biosphere and the use of existing substrates and most probably processes. After all, the basic idea, at least with reference to synthetic xenobiology is to achieve biotechnological effects and massive, expansive applications without the dangers of genetic/genomic pollution.

3. **Low compatibility**

It refers rather to the realm of exobiology, with non-carbon biochemistries that allow no material common ground, but there could be analogues between the

Box 4.2 contd. ...

...Box 4.2 contd.

functionality and the engineering infrastructure of the alien and common life physiologies. For example, the existence of coding macromolecules informing the production of effector catalytic molecules through successive generations is a functional concept that may be applied to non-carbon biochemistries, but the coding elements cannot be processed in any way by the different enzymes implicated in the different steps of coding, preservation, transmission and translation of the nucleic acid genetics.

4.   Null compatibility

This refers to lifeforms based on different basic molecules and wholly different procedures. A Sci-Fi example here could be crystals of different elements as their development satisfies some prerogatives of life, including the creation of higher order out of lower-ordered materials and coding of information in introducing abnormalities in the crystal structure. Alternatively, biochemistries based on completely different basic molecules, such as SiO-SiO or Si-Si chain macromolecules, could have created alternative lifeforms especially in different environmental conditions of temperature, pressure or atmosphere composition. Such entities would pray on the inorganic environment, would not directly interact biochemically with the biosphere elements and would thus pose no threat of genetic pollution or interbreeding. This does not exclude *a priori* similar mechanisms and procedures, but the material base of their physiology is incompatible with the basic elements and biomolecules constituting life in the earth's biosphere. It must be stressed that lifeforms as these may come from exoworlds but also from the shadow biosphere of the earth. It would be the object of cosmobiology as a whole, for it falls within the scope of astro-, exo- and xenobiology, albeit with conditions in each case.

---

but not restricted to antisepsis, asepsia and sterilization) are applicable. For example, even if the acting macromolecules are proteins containing other amino acids, or molecules entirely different from the known peptides, they would still be arranged in 3-D by secondary chemical bonds, albeit different ones; thus, they would be sensitive to factors detrimental for such bonds. The biochemistry of such (micro)organisms may work on very different pH and temperature levels, but changes in pH and temperature would still be impactful for the survival of such organisms and the integrity of their physiology.

Genetic pollution

The spotlight fell on genetic pollution for the first time with the advent of GMOs for environmental applications (Sirohi et al. 2014, Diwo and Budisa 2018), originally in agriculture but subsequently in forestry/environment, microbiome engineering and shaping, and the use of custom-made biologicals for dietary and therapeutic applications. Genetic pollution is a quantitative rather than qualitative concept. Highly heterologous reshuffling of DNA happens spontaneously in nature, the uptake of host sequences by viruses during transduction being a first step, and the uptake of naked DNA from bacteria during the transformation procedure being the main event. By making massive amounts of synthesized/engineered sequences available in a wide range of environments as eDNA/environmental DNA, a term meant to signify a more inclusive and diverse range of sequences, not only naked (Colnaghi et al. 2020) at spatio-temporal coincidence with diverse microbiomes, the quantitative dimension becomes qualitative. Such multifaceted abundance greatly multiplies the evolutionary throughput of natural environments and microbiomes and is bound to kick-start the emergence of novel microorganisms quite unpredictably in terms of extent, impact and volume (Gillings and Stokes 2012). Of course, genetic pollution does not apply strictly to eDNA. Other forms or conditions of DNA also qualify, even without transient participation in the eDNA pool, at least as the latter is understood *sensu stricto*, that is, DNA without capsid/membrane sheath. Heterologous pollination, viral transduction between highly diverse species and other forms of lateral and vertical gene transfer may also qualify for genetic pollution if the expected results are predominantly detrimental in terms of impact or volume or both.

The emergence of novel microorganisms transcends the conventional view of the microbiome. It is plausible that it may lead to different macroorganisms if the concept of the holobiont describes a more integrated set of interactions and interdependence between hosts and microbiomes than we understand today (Richardson 2017). Science fiction has repeatedly explored the transformation of macro-hosts due to microsymbionts, usually alien in nature and origin. Although this is beyond current scientific substantiation, it lies within the horizon of possible.

The factuality of more kinds of DNA sequences, more massively available and in highly dispersed environments almost concurrently, under intense exchange of matter (mainly but not exclusively through trade and travel) means that the probability of an evolutionary event detrimental in impact is much higher than the occurrence of an improved model. The maths describing it would be a welcome improvement on planetary biosecurity. Even without such maths readily available, it follows—a bitter lesson from COVID-19—that timely containment after a risk factor is detected and identified as a threat, is out of the question.

It can be concluded that genetic pollution is subject to genomic compatibility, but this should be interpreted *sensu lato*; the obvious issue is microorganisms using the known nucleic acids and with a similar genetic code. If different genetic codes are used in some xenobiote, these may be *interpreted* in some of the known ones, should some structural degradation of the carrier be implementable. A natural analogue here is the Thymine-Uracil duet, both of which pair with Adenine. If similar patterns are applicable to the xenobiote code, then its sequences would produce evolutionary material, although not predictably; the traits of the xenoorganism will not be transplanted to the receiver of the xenosequences, but novel sequences will be introduced—translatable if suitably integrated, according to Chance (in terms of Open Reading Frames and genomic position) and the translational mechanism of the said receiver, that is, the version of the genetic code it abides to. Different receiving organisms of the exact same sequence in the exact same or equivalent genomic spot may produce different proteins due to slight differences in the genetic code.

Synthetic Xenobiology as a potential liability or risk factor

The notion of xenobiology has been officially differentiated from alien/estranged organisms, irrespective of their origin and physiology, to comprise advances including but not limited to synthetic biology (Unknown n.d. c). Thus, at the conceptual level, the engineered (micro)organisms that differ significantly from the ones encountered in the biosphere have been added to the category of xenoorganisms.

The 'significantly' clause needs some more elaboration. It refers not to form (morphophenotype), and definitely not to the use of standard metabolites in input or output, although both sources and products may well be much more diverse and perhaps different; however, that cannot be a defining issue as the reason for developing many synthetic organisms is to fulfil biotechnological niches, both existing (in biosphere and industry) and completely novel, which is acceptable only for the latter (Atlas 1988, Dapurkar and Telang 2017, Janatunaim and Fibriani 2020). The main difference though is in the realm of *throughput*, where one or more levels of the mechanism are 'significantly' different. This significance implies the impossibility of any natural (through evolution) development of similar (not analogous) molecules in the normal horizon of events. The most important and perhaps defining level is the genomic/genetic. A coding system based on a notion of nucleic acids but differing in form and internal function (differences in the structure and perhaps in the number of code letters) makes the informational exchange with the members of the biosphere impossible. This introduces the xenonucleic acids (XNAs) as a quintessential failsafe in this concept (Schmidt 2010, Acevedo-Rocha and Budisa 2016, Diwo and Budisa 2018, Gómez-Tatay and Hernández-Andreu 2019).

The use of proteins and other metabolites may be identical, similar or once more 'significantly' dissimilar. Herein, an example can be found in biocatalytic biomolecules of different natures, including but not restricted to foldamers (Acevedo-Rocha and Budisa 2016) instead of the enzyme-ribozyme range available ·in the biosphere (Völler and Budisa 2017, Sadler et al. 2021). A less significant alteration would be enzymes and ribozymes made of amino acids and ribonucleotides different from the existing ones. These should not necessarily be currently unknown/non-existent; they may be some existing ones not currently participating in the formation of such macromolecules. These monomers, different from but chemically similar to the ones actually used as building blocks, may represent a portion of the macromolecule's sequence, combined with the standard ones (Diwo and Budisa 2018, Gómez-Tatay and Hernández-Andreu 2019); or they may make up the sequence *in toto*, fully substituting the current ones (Figure 4.3).

The design of novel biomolecules made up of the existing building blocks, meaning a recombination or reshuffle of sorts, would most probably not qualify for 'significant', but this may need further elaboration. It is actually within the realm of standard evolution and biochemical and genetic engineering as the basic ingredients are the same and there is no firewall between natural organisms and the engineered ones. With this background, there is a subtle spin-off: if the bases and the code remain identical but the backbone changes (Figure 4.4) along with the involved pathways for the production of the monomers and the elongation of the chains, this IS a firewall

Xenobiology categories

- Xenonucleic Acids-
difference in backbone (HNA, TNA, CeNA, PNA et.c)
OR arsenate instead of phosphate

- Irregular Nucleic Acids
difference in the bases

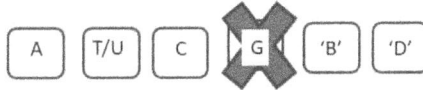

A | T/U | C | G | 'B' | 'D'

- Xenoproteins/xenoribozymes
Other AAs/rNMPs

- Xenocatalytes
No AAs/rNMPs   and/or other conformations (Foldamers)

Figure 4.3. The different levels of xenobiotic differentiation in biomolecules.

between the engineered and the natural realms. One such natural case is that of organisms using Arsenic-*As* instead of Phosphorus-P (arsenate instead of phosphate) in their nucleic acids, as mentioned above, although it remains controversial whether this is an alternate and not an exclusive pathway (Wolfe-Simon et al. 2011, Check Hayden 2012). The substitution of pentose sugar (ribose/deoxyribose) by some exose or any other non-sugar element seems to receive much more attention though (Schmidt 2010).

The idea behind synthetic xenobiology is usually thought to be the absolute negation of genetic pollution issues (Schmidt 2010, Acevedo-Rocha and Budisa 2016, Diwo and Budisa 2018). Coupled with self-evident auxotrophy (Schmidt 2010, Acevedo-Rocha and Budisa 2016, Völler and Budisa 2017, Gómez-Tatay

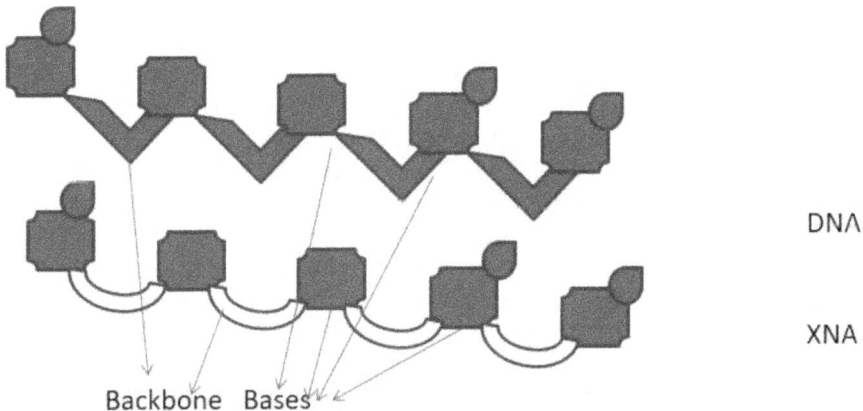

DNA

XNA

Backbone   Bases

Figure 4.4. DNA and XNA have identical coding elements—i.e., the bases, but differ in the support element, i.e., the backbone. Usual differences refer to the sugar being substituted by another organic moiety, or the phosphate being replaced by another element (arsenate for instance).

and Hernández-Andreu 2019) as the functional biomolecules are 'significantly' different from existing analogues, this supposedly tackles the issue of biosecurity as well. These organisms with their special needs cannot survive outside controlled environments. However, there are two fundamental issues in this simple and short paragraph:

The first is that the idea of xenobiology, or rather xenomicrobiology (Acevedo-Rocha and Budisa 2016), was *not* conceived to reduce the danger of genetic pollution, but to introduce really proprietary elements in the biotech industry. The proprietary status claimed by many firms for natural organisms (Balachandra Nair and Ramachandranna 2010) and even for engineered strains based on natural ones may, in the future, be claimed void by regulatory authorities less inclined towards corporate interests. The fact that something made available freely is actually hijacked and propertied by some concern, simply because it described, purified or declared it first, reminds of the Gold Fever Laws, which do not appeal to many non-corporate concerns, especially citizens and pre-industrialist cultures. But with something developed from a clean sheet, no one may have objections and even less so when this course would really weaken the demands and claims of the usual biotechnological concerns, basing their efforts on partially or wholly natural organisms (Cooper 1983, Balachandra Nair and Ramachandranna 2010, Sekar and Kandavel 2019). A convention for the Rights of the Organisms is expected at some time to regulate or deregulate the biotechnological industry domain, and the synthetic xenobiology in this context seems a mixed blessing. Allegedly it came to moderate the negative effects on the industry of concerns and developments as the above. But it might just as well precipitate this kind of effects and thus create an opportunity for the few within a crisis for the many.

The flip side in this story of enterprising proactive security is that the whole mechanism—from the blueprints to the final effectors—could be proprietary and known only to the developing authority, possibly protected against analysis by corporate-friendly and copyrights legislation. This means that in case something goes amiss, at any level (from reshuffling some native microbiomes to starting epidemics in cultures/cultivations and breeding stocks or communities), there is no way to analyze the xenoorganism for detecting, diagnosing and predicting vulnerabilities and liabilities. Not by the normal procedure of genomic and metagenomic scanning and metabolome or proteome analysis, possibly not even with structural analyses using imaging or spectroscopy (Velegraki and Zerva 2020). Only crude functional inroads may be readily implementable. Thus, in the case of accidental, perpetrated or any other conceivable illicit use of xenoorganisms, the responding authorities will be faced with something literally alien, as its nature along with the coding of the respective genetic blueprint will be initially unknown. Taking into consideration the time needed to resolve the structure of SARS-CoV2, this makes any comparison look bleak at the very least, not to mention the actual translation of such a resolution to actionable results.

The second issue is that in order to exploit such on-demand microorganisms where it would matter the most, i.e., in the open environment (Diwo and Budisa 2018), for purposes such as land reclaim, bioremediation, terraforming, waste management/decomposition/biodegradation, biofuel production, ore enrichment, microbiome shaping, etc., they *are* to be made to operate independently, without auxotrophies. Their proprietary systems would have interfaces to produce the necessary biomolecules from organic or inorganic raw materials (Völler and Budisa 2017). This exploitation scheme is the most interesting and lucrative one and it is a given that it will be, sooner rather than later, authorized—not only to recuperate the original massive investments in technology development, but also because the market share would be significant compared to, for example, the use for medical purposes, in the guise of 'xenobiologicals/xenobiopharmaceuticals'. Thus, the safety precaution, in terms of biosecurity and not of genetic pollution, is conditional and of a very limited prospective application in temporal and circumstantial terms.

Existing microorganisms and perhaps compounds may still have a detrimental and even lethal effect on xenobiological organisms, but this is speculative—they may not. Should the xeno-epitopes be of constitution allowing no electrochemical attachment to the existing paratopes (Akbar et al. 2021), despite possible structural compatibility, no antibody-mediated intervention—from immune response to serodiagnostics (Coelho et al. 2015, Haake and Zückert 2018)—may be applicable. Harder shells, such as calcium-containing linings over or inserts within the cellular envelope, would negate the direct complement inactivation by perforation of the cell envelope/membrane (Fishelson and Kirschfink 2019). Ultimately, even if not designed as dual-use agents, synthetic Xenobiota may follow particular and peculiar meta-evolutionary pathways and turn into biothreats in a stochastic manner, while the expected volume of their use, qualitative and quantitative, is prone to be the ultimate risk enhancer (Gibson et al. 2010).

References

Acevedo-Rocha, C.G. and Budisa, N. (2016). Xenomicrobiology: A roadmap for genetic code engineering. Microbial Biotechnology, 9(5): 666–676. doi: 10.1111/1751-7915.12398.

Aguilar, W. et al. (2014). The past, present, and future of artificial life. Front Robot AI, 1(8). doi: 10.3389/frobt.2014.00008.

Akbar, R. et al. (2021). A compact vocabulary of paratope-epitope interactions enables predictability of antibody-antigen binding. Cell Reports, 34(11): 108856. doi: 10.1016/J.CELREP.2021.108856.

Atlas, R.M. (1988). Biodegradation of hydrocarbons in the environment. Basic Life Sciences, 45: 211–222. doi: 10.1007/978-1-4899-0824-7_14.

Balachandra Nair, R. and Ramachandranna, P.C. (2010). Patenting of microorganisms: Systems and concerns. Journal of Commercial Biotechnology, 16(4): 337–347. doi: 10.1057/JCB.2010.20.

Budisa, N. et al. (2020). Xenobiology: A Journey towards Parallel Life Forms. ChemBioChem, 21(16): 2228–2231. doi: 10.1002/CBIC.202000141

Check Hayden, E. (2012). Study challenges existence of arsenic-based life. Nature on line. doi: 10.1038/NATURE.2012.9861.

Cleland, C.E. and Copley, S.D. (2005). The possibility of alternative microbial life on Earth. International Journal of Astrobiology, 4(3-4): 165–173. doi: 10.1017/S147355040500279X.

Cleland, C.E. (2007). Epistemological issues in the study of microbial life: alternative terran biospheres? Studies in History and Philosophy of Biological and Biomedical Sciences, 38(4): 847–861. doi: 10.1016/J.SHPSC.2007.09.007.

Coelho, E.A.F. et al. (2015). Theranostic applications of phage display to control leishmaniasis: Selection of biomarkers for serodiagnostics, vaccination, and immunotherapy. Revista da Sociedade Brasileira de Medicina Tropical, 48(4): 370–379. doi: 10.1590/0037-8682-0096-2015.

Colnaghi, M. et al. (2020). Genome expansion in early eukaryotes drove the transition from lateral gene transfer to meiotic sex. Elife, 9: 1–16. doi: 10.7554/ELIFE.58873.

Cooper, A. (1983). Patentability of genetically engineered microorganisms. JAMA: The Journal of the American Medical Association, 249(12): 1553–4.

Croom, E. (2012). Metabolism of xenobiotics of human environments. pp. 31–88. *In*: Hodgson, E. (ed.). Progress in Molecular Biology and Translational Science. Academic Press. doi: 10.1016/B978-0-12-415813-9.00003-9.

Dapurkar, D. and Telang, M. (2017). A patent landscape on application of microorganisms in construction industry. World Journal of Microbiology & Biotechnology, 33(7). doi: 10.1007/S11274-017-2302-X.

Davidson, R.A. (1985). Immunology of parasitic infections. The Medical clinics of North America, 69(4): 751–758. doi: 10.1016/S0025-7125(16)31017-3.

Diwo, C. and Budisa, N. (2018). Alternative biochemistries for alien life: Basic concepts and requirements for the design of a robust biocontainment system in genetic isolation. Genes, 10(1). doi: 10.3390/genes10010017.

Fishelson, Z. and Kirschfink, M. (2019). Complement C5b-9 and cancer: Mechanisms of cell damage, cancer counteractions, and approaches for intervention. Frontiers in Immunology, 10. doi: 10.3389/FIMMU.2019.00752.

Foster, K.R. et al. (2017). The evolution of the host microbiome as an ecosystem on a leash. Nature, 548(7665): 43–51.

Gibson, D.G. et al. (2010). Creation of a bacterial cell controlled by a chemically synthesized genome. Science, 329(5987): 52–56. doi: 10.1126/science.1190719.

Gillings, M.R. and Stokes, H.W. (2012). Are humans increasing bacterial evolvability? Trends in Ecology & Evolution, 27(6): 346–352. doi: 10.1016/J.TREE.2012.02.006.

Gómez-Tatay, L. and Hernández-Andreu, J.M. (2019). Biosafety and biosecurity in synthetic biology: A review. Critical Reviews in Environmental Science and Technology, 49(17): 1587–1621. doi: 10.1080/10643389.2019.1579628.

Haake, D.A. and Zückert, W.R. (2018). Spirochetal lipoproteins in pathogenesis and immunity. Current Topics in Microbiology and Immunology, 415: 239–271. doi: 10.1007/82_2017_78.

Janatunaim, R.Z. and Fibriani, A. (2020). Construction and cloning of plastic-degrading recombinant enzymes (MHETase). Recent Patents on Biotechnology, 14(3): 229–234. doi: 10.2174/1872208314666200311104541.

McKay, C.P. (2010). An origin of life on Mars. Cold Spring Harbor Perspectives in Biology, 2(4). doi: 10.1101/CSHPERSPECT.A003509.

NASA (no date) a: https://astrobiology.nasa.gov/about/history-of-astrobiology/

NASA (no date) b: https://astrobiology.nasa.gov/nai/annual-reports/2005/ucla/geobiology-and-the-geochemistry-of-early-earth/index.html.

NASA (no date) c: https://exoplanets.nasa.gov/what-is-an-exoplanet/overview/.

NASA (no date) d: https://astrobiology.nasa.gov/research/astrobiology-at-nasa/exobiology/.

Obeng, N. et al. (2021). Evolution of microbiota–host associations: The microbe's perspective. Trends in Microbiology, 29(9): 779–787. doi: 10.1016/J.TIM.2021.02.005.

Palmer, M. et al. (2017). On defining global catastrophic biological risks. Health Security, 15(4): 347–348. doi: 10.1089/HS.2017.0057.

Richardson, L.A. (2017). Evolving as a holobiont. PLoS Biology, 15(2). doi: 10.1371/JOURNAL.PBIO.2002168.

Sadler, J.C. et al. (2021).Interfacing non-enzymatic catalysis with living microorganisms. RSC Chemical Biology, 2(4): 1073–1083. doi: 10.1039/D1CB00072A.

Schmidt, M. (2010). Xenobiology: A new form of life as the ultimate biosafety tool. Bioessays, 32(4): 322–331. doi: 10.1002/bies.200900147.

Schmidt, M., Pei, L. and Budisa, N. (2018). Xenobiology: State-of-the-art, ethics, and philosophy of new-to-nature organisms. Advances in Biochemical Engineering/Biotechnology, 162: 301–316. doi: 10.1007/10_2016_14.

Schulman, R. and Winfree, E. (2008). How crystals that sense and respond to their environments could evolve. Natural Computing, 7: 219–237. doi: 10.1007/s11047-007-9046-8.

Schulze-Makuch, D. and Irwin, L.N. (2006). The prospect of alien life in exotic forms on other worlds.Die Naturwissenschaften. Naturwissenschaften, 93(4): 155–172. doi: 10.1007/S00114-005-0078-6.

Schulze-Makuch, D. et al. (2017). The adaptability of life on Earth and the diversity of planetary habitats. Frontiers in Microbiology. doi: 10.3389/FMICB.2017.02011.

Sekar, S. and Kandavel, D. (2019). Patenting of microorganisms. Encyclopedia of Microbiology. Academic Press, pp. 426–442. doi: 10.1016/B978-0-12-809633-8.13086-9.

Sirohi, S. et al. (2014). Genetic pollution and biodiversity. International Journal of Recent Scientific Research, 5(6): 1639–1642.

Unknown (no date) a: https://socratic.org/questions/what-are-the-differences-between-astrobiology-exobiology-and-xenobiology).

Unknown (no date) b: https://wikidiff.com/astrobiology/xenobiology.

Unknown (no date) c: https://en.wikipedia.org/wiki/Xenobiology.

Velegraki, A. and Zerva, L. (2020). Identifying microbiota: Genomic, mass-spectrometric, and serodiagnostic approaches. pp. 77–94. *In*: Kambouris, M. and Velegraki, A. (eds.). Microbiomics: Dimensions, Applications and Translational Implications of Human and Environmental Microbiome Research. ELSEVIER ACADEMIC PRESS.

Völler, J.S. and Budisa, N. (2017). Coupling genetic code expansion and metabolic engineering for synthetic cells. Current Opinion in Biotechnology. Elsevier Ltd, pp. 1–7. doi: 10.1016/j.copbio.2017.02.002.

Wolfe-Simon, F. et al. (2011). A bacterium that can grow by using arsenic instead of phosphorus. Science, 332(6034), pp. 1163–1166. doi: 10.1126/SCIENCE.1197258.

Yokoyama, W.M. and Colonna, M. (2008). Innate immunity to pathogens. Current Opinion in Immunology, 20(1): 1. doi: 10.1016/J.COI.2008.01.004.

5

Nature Avenging

Manousos E. Kambouris,[1] Aristea Velegraki[2] and George P. Patrinos[3],*

Introduction

Infectious diseases seem to be back with a vengeance rather than becoming gradually extinct, as was the prevailing view in the last quarter of the 20th century—a very potent reminder of the correctness of 'views' and 'projections' of experts, especially in the biomedical sector. The COVID-19 pandemic underlined the conclusion that infectious diseases will still plague, if not outright doom, humanity, and actually the humanome, the latter defined as an inclusive concept (Kambouris et al. 2018) encompassing all the species domesticated or otherwise depending on humanity for their current survival status (mostly plants cultivated and livestock bred). It is obvious that there are anthropogenic and non-anthropogenic, spontaneous reasons for such a dramatic comeback, which refers to both qualitative and quantitative parameters. Larger populations from more microbial species become more virulent and/or pathogenic, and occasionally also resistant to antimicrobials like antibiotics.

All of this should be considered from a very different, actually expansive, perspective. Although Nature is still not recognized by Science as a cognitive entity, with any pretense or intention to act or react, for better or worse, it is understood to

[1] University of Patras, School of Health Sciences, Department of Pharmacy, Patras, Greece & The Golden Helix Foundation, London, United Kingdom.
Email: mekambouris@yahoo.com, ORCID iD: https://orcid.org/0000-0002-3205-4797
[2] Medical School, National and Kapodistrian University of Athens, Athens, Greece & Bioiatriki SA, Athens, Greece.
Email: aveleg@med.uoa.gr, ORCID iD: https://orcid.org/0000-0002-7605-0210
[3] University of Patras, School of Health Sciences, Department of Pharmacy, Patras, Greece & United Arab Emirates University, College of Medicine and Health Sciences, Department of Genetics and Genomics, & Zayed Center for Health Sciences, Al-Ain, Abu Dhabi, UAE.
* Corresponding author: gpatrinos@upatras.gr, ORCID iD: https://orcid.org /0000-0002-0519-7776

involve a complex set of balance, counterbalance and adaptational networks that may be considered to create response or reaction; response is not a valid concept in this context, but reaction *is*. It clearly refers to the events unfolding through deterministic automation—complex to the point of unpredictability, but still deterministic in many cases. The possibility to quantify enormous numbers of complex variables as pitched by the Quantified Planet (Özdemir 2018) suggests the multi-aspect examination of the natural world, especially the living entities. The compartmentalization of previous generations of scientists, handy if one is to define areas of study and apply different sets of research principles, was optimized by faculty; it has sown its limits though and is plighted by many limitations. It is obsolete and inapplicable in any effort to achieve a breakthrough. The burst in microbiome applications (and studies) is a direct consequence of new technologies, made up partly or wholly by the direct and indirect results of the explosive progress in IT, especially in the sectors pertaining to biotechnology and bioscience. Starting with single-cell genomics (Paolillo et al. 2019) and metagenomics (Wooley et al. 2010, Laurence 2020), all the way to the concepts of microbiomes (Kambouris and Velegraki 2020), holobionts (Bordenstein and Theis 2015) and the exogenome as a prospective aspect of environmental DNA/eDNA (Kambouris et al. 2018), integration in different levels does follow the trends of Information Technology (IT)—nothing mystical, at least nothing self-evidently so, and nothing malicious either. And what we may apperceive as Nature's reaction would be obviously shaped somehow similarly, although the specifics cannot be foretold, at least not yet. Forecast is a somewhat imprecise science, the projections of climate change/crisis being a valuable lesson on the subject (Perry 2019). Calculations in the context of more-than-Tera-Big Data may someday change that, but this is a long way into the future.

The hidden nature

The mainstream idea has long been that evolution progresses from the simpler to the more complicated, thus prokaryota pre-date eukaryota. At some point, the eukaryota developed enough to create multicellular organisms (Trigos et al. 2018, Márquez-Zacarías et al. 2021). The existing forms are snapshots of evolution; other forms were dead ends and still others were superseded by the more evolved models in the depth of time—especially their evolved descendants which competed for the same niche and habitat. However, since not all prokaryota became eukaryota, the ones not taking this step kept on evolving and may produce new versions of cell evolution that may duplicate previous pedigrees, or result in something new.

There is an understandable consensus that size and complexity are associated (Bonner 2004): to support size, which essentially allows economies of scale, a more efficient way of management is required. Compartmentalization, division of tasks and optimized oversight and control allocate the given resources better than the less elaborate arrangements. They are prone to disruption, deregulation and systemic failure—a reason for the smaller prokaryota (simpler, more resilient and robust) to be colonizers of extreme environments. As a result, the mainstream version is that the better and efficient arrangement of the eukaryota is needed for large cells, with their efficiently located and organized genome keeping track of a more efficient, differentiated, advanced and dedicated biochemical machinery. Multicellularity demands even more elaborate mechanisms, both in terms of procedures and parts/ molecules, given that communication has to extend to transcellular level in order to synchronize different cells; thus, signaling systems must be evolved, produced, maintained and, of course, coded—all at a great expense of energy. As a result, even more elaborate and efficient genomes are needed than for a unicellular eukaryote. Ultimately, the apex is the differentiated multicellular organism, with different cell types according to position (tissues) or time (ontogenesis), for which *differential* command signals and responses are needed.

This scheme is straightforward and logical; however, it is at the very least oversimplified. Different mechanistic solutions have been developed and they are successful in functional terms, as evident from the current, living examples.

Evolution

It seems that a very large single-cell size is not a prerogative for an eukaryote, as presupposed with the paradigm of the neuron in mind; the same goes for multicellularity: the cases of actinobacteria, *Streptomyces* and *Nocardia* are perfect examples. The highly ordered successive division patterns shown mostly by *Sarcina* spp. (Canale-Parola and Wolfe 1960, Begg and Donachie 1998) point to the same conclusion, without even mentioning the concept of the germ-ganism (Kambouris et al. 2022). Actually, prokaryota seem perfectly capable of becoming complex cells or organisms, as in developing long fibrils, with linear succession and vertical septa individualizing each cell, perfectly analogous to septate hyphae in higher fungal taxa. The septal formation excludes the possibility of simple linear aggregation and requires the concession of multicellular status, for the septa are evidently different than two touching or even fused cell envelopes as obvious in images (Volland et al. 2022).

Regarding the former attestation, size matters and so do some infrastructures necessary to develop and maintain the increased size and volume. As cell size increases, so do energy demands, but the volume-to-surface ratio becomes important in prokaryota, as the inner surface of the cell membrane is the signature bench for many a biochemical reaction, including respiration. Extended membranic formations, with dense folds, is the eukaryotic solution to the problem, providing ample surface for biochemical reactions, including translation and protein synthesis of much higher efficiency, for the membrane support allows elaborate processing. Thus, the equivalent of the inner membranes of mitochondria and of the endoplasmic reticulum are needed to support large cell volumes and masses; these may be extensions of the plasma membrane folded inwards and possibly even twisted to offer compartmentalization of sorts. This solution allows a primitive nucleus—one or more copies of the prokaryotic genome in a membranous compartment, tied to a specific spot of the cell (Volland et al. 2022). This strict location allows spatially limited and well-defined protein production at a core spot. The spatial limitations increase the efficiency, and multiple such cores within the cell create a dispersed pattern of translation which, in a stable environment with few needs to adapt to changing conditions, may support large cell sizes, even in the absence of one of the key eukaryotic characteristics that support large cell sizes, i.e., the elaborate intracellular transportation systems, implemented especially by microtubules. Thus, the eukaryota have advanced mechanisms of deterministic and adaptable intracellular transportation, which optimize the spatial efficiency of all processes, despite chance phenomena. This *is* a prerogative for the combination of processes in different biocompartments in a coherent and coordinated way. In prokaryota, chance motion is expected to place the different ingredients into actionable distance from each other at some time, and this is expedited by limited volumes and short distances. The eukaryote recreates this short-distance effect by compartmentalization, which also adds a twist—only the molecules needed for a certain process or group of processes are aggregated in such compartments, thus reducing the possibility of cross-reactions and interference, while all necessary items are constantly in close proximity and occasionally in optimized spatial distribution; in Golgi tanks and mitochondria for instance. All of the above require diverse and intense protein synthesis to develop and maintain the enzymatic systems needed for uprated metabolism, and for the formation and maintenance of the compartmentalization—physical as well as functional. This obviously requires better organization and regulation, impossible without an advanced arrangement of the genomic information, which would allow great saving capacity in small space, enhanced by increased reliability in fidelity, protection and restoration of the genomic data. The efficient duplication of code records, especially for propagation, is of vital importance.

But the primary issue is the mechanism of selective retrieval and expression of coding units, which allows differential access of the expression machinery to the genomic elements, thus allowing for reshaping expression networks and consequently different forms and functions of the cells, a prerogative for the ontogenetic process. The advent of nucleus, with selective access to the genome and the steady location of both the DNA and all the enzymes necessary for its proper function, does much to this direction, but the arrangement of the DNA in chromosomes, very efficiently packaged and arranged in separate volumes of the genome library, is just as important and the similar multipartite genome in some Prokarya (diCenzo and Finan 2017) underlines said importance. In fact, the nucleus as understood currently would not be possible without the chromosome revolution, which allows on-demand condensation and relaxation of the chromatin in a predictable manner, so as to allow optimal function and also efficient and reliable duplication and segregation during cell division. Nucleoforming, especially in the autogenous model (Devos et al. 2014, Hendrickson and Poole 2018), is *the* transition from the pokaryote condition to the eukaryote by definition. It is to be followed by compartmentalization—the formation of different membranous organelles and the increase in size, the latter supported by a novel, high-capacity transportation and transformation system(s). The addition of mitochondria and plastids is almost certainly attributable to an endosymbiotic model (Hendrickson and Poole 2018), but the nucleoformation not convincingly so.

Thus, to evolve from unicellular prokaroyta to multicellular eukaryota, there are more options than the obvious linear one: first, a step to proto-eukaryota like *Giardia lamblia*, with (most probably autogenously) properly formed nucleus (actually nuclei) and microtubules, but only a few organelles (Svärd et al. 2003), and then to the fully evolved unicellular eukaryota, complete with large ribosomes and diverse membranous organelles, plus mitochondria and occasionally plastids, acquired under an endosymbiotic model (Hendrickson and Poole 2018). An alternative path may have been the multicellular prokaryota, of typical cell size but multicellular organization—typical or atypical (germ-ganisms)—and the gigantocells, directly reminiscent of macroorganisms in nature and size, but unicellular and prokaryote in structure; perhaps prokaryotic syncytia. Whether these phases are divergent from a linear succession of evolutionary events or were somehow incorporated in a more complex, non-linear evolutionary tract remains a valid issue begging study; it also transcends more fundamental evolutionary queries (Cleland and Copley 2005). The gigantic macroorganismic bacteria are an evolutionary link that may explain the steps of the original evolution on earth (Volland et al. 2022). Perhaps superimposed evolutionary courses may be understood (Hendrickson and Poole 2018) as another association after the divergent and convergent ones. The 'superimposed' version should be understood as similar regarding the evolutionary dimension, but on a different level, meaning that the processes occurred in different timelines, following non-simultaneous or non-concurrent courses, in contrast to 'parallel' evolutionary pathways, which are understood as occurring in the same temporal context, although not necessarily in the same spatial one.

The emergence process(es)

The issue of emerging pathogens has been undeniably hot for quite some time and there has been constant talk, along with an increasing stream of publications long before the COVID-19 pandemic and also before the steady arrival of emerging viral pathogens that have infested the world since 2010 or so. The establishment of the term "emerging" is sourced to a US document regarding future biothreats, the HSPD-18 (*Homeland Security Presidential Directive/HSPD-18-Medical Countermeasures Against Weapons of Mass Destruction* 2007); the latter are categorized into 4 groups, the first being the original agents, prominent amongst which are the Dirty Dozen (Cieslak et al. 2018). The second group is that of emerging pathogens and refers to the only one of the truly future threat areas (unidentified as yet) without direct evolutionary human involvement. The other two groups, the enhanced and the advanced pathogens, refer to different degrees of manipulation; the former refers to the existing agents enhanced by tampering, and the latter to the engineering of completely new agents (Colf 2016). A newer classification recently proposed for biothreats (Kambouris 2021a), suggesting six generations of bioagents, follows the essence of the original 4-level system in the distinction of the enhanced and the advanced agents as generations 2 and 3 respectively, but elaborates the latter further, as it segregates genomic attack agents, bioregulators/ biotoxins, xenobiological constructs and hybrid techno-bioagents. Moreover, in the newer classification, the group of emerging pathogens is not afforded any special status as in case of the previous one (Colf 2016). Regardless of the reason for their delayed arrival, emerging pathogens are natural products and thus basically subject to standard limitations and thus part of the 1st generation of bioagents in terms of biodefense/biosecurity (Colf 2016, Kambouris 2021a).

Irrespective of their status from a biosecurity viewpoint, the emerging pathogens have posed problems far before they were named as such, and, thus, understanding their extreme diversity even on the subject of their emergence is quintessential to deliberate responses and attempt projections. A novel pathogen may emerge in several ways in a pathogenic capacity. First, an entirely new organism with pathogenic traits may appear in a new spatio-temporal continuum (physical emergence). An entirely new microbiote, somehow finding its way and becoming an opportunistic or mandatory pathogen, meaning that there are one or more naïve or at least susceptible host populations. It is a structural change, for something entirely new appears (Kambouris 2021a).

The other possibility is that the new pathogen, once more qualifying for one or more given susceptible population/species, has not appeared *de novo*, but has been there in a different, benign capacity. It suddenly starts behaving aggressively and carries different and additional traits that endow it with virulence—a concept christened "gain of function" in a very polite and politically correct manner, usually referring to such events of human agency and engineering (Dance 2021). This case—evolutionary emergence—is an absolute functional change as there are new functions inserted into the existing players. The expansion of the concept in existing pathogens becoming more virulent suggests the idea of the superpathogen *sensu lato* (Kambouris 2021a).

The third possibility (functional emergence) is that an existing organism has not changed in its basic physiological realities, but the wider environmental changes recast it with a pathogenic potential, as dynamic balances among different species and niches reboot in a fast-changing environment, the latter taken *sensu lato*. It is a relatively functional change (Kambouris 2021a).

The above trident of spontaneous threat development is comprehensively examined herein. It must be stressed that accidental events of human agency are included (this qualifies as the revenge and chastising of Mother Nature to the arrogant and selfish human kind), but perpetrated events and risk factors explicitly engineered to any degree—from microbiome engineering and organism engineering by synthetic biology to intentional dispersion of potentially harmful strains—refer to a very different group of events and is detailed in a separate chapter. Although, superficially, the intention is only a detail of minor importance in the philosophy and science of infectious threats, it is the most important detail, for it entails the existence of an adversary intelligence, indicating towards an effort to optimize and to mask intentions, facts and procedures—in other words, prospective and retrospective counters—to hinder the response efforts by the responders and the respective institutions, organisms and authorities.

1. Physical emergence and de novo appearance

The appearance of novel agents refers to an evolutionary tract, of course, that was followed and implemented outside the effects of the concerned continuum; on the contrary, the evolutionary events that have occurred during (and mostly due to) the concerned spatio-temporal and factual continuum are dealt with in the next part.

The most straightforward case is definitely the occurrence of new and spontaneously evolved microorganisms, as they feature from the standard procedures of natural selection, *without* the direct or indirect intervention of human activity in any sense. Especially hot and humid environments with plenty of biomass are factories of evolution due to the high population densities that increase the stochastic potential for evolution, while also constituting the selection mechanism through fierce inter- and intra-species competition for plentiful in volume but spatially scarce resources (Hibbing et al. 2010, Ghoul and Mitri 2016). Such areas are not relevant only to wildlife, thus needing a translocation/transportation step to cause an epidemic. Humanome interfaces are essential (Lovgren 2003, Temmam et al. 2022); especially with highly diverse wildlife (Magouras et al. 2020) and, in many cases, in social units with little regard for biosecurity and biovigilance and bereft of equipment and training for both prospective and retrospective agent control. From such interfaces, microorganisms presenting threat features for human hosts or the humanome in general, may be routed to their new host environments by chance due to the massive evolutionary output where they may encounter new hosts, to colonize and later plight while adaptation steps expand the new host basis to multiple species or other host taxa (Sharma and Chakrabarti 2020, Sharma et al. 2021). It must be noted that multi-species hosting does not necessarily focus on similar taxa; in many cases, wildly different species may be hosts for extremely aggressive pathogens, the diversity occasionally extending to kingdoms if not domains (Van Baarlen et al. 2007, Batista et al. 2020).

In the context of diverse host bases, the avian flu with immense human toll in epidemics is one easily understood case; actually, though, the opportunistic human/animal pathogens that are originally encountered as plant pathogens, must always be borne in mind. Different *Aspergillus* and *Fusarium* molds may cause mayhem in animal populations under some conditions, whether biological, like immunodeficiencies, or ecological, like the reduced thermal buffering between the host and the pathogen (Sharma and Chakrabarti 2020). Non-septic complications such as allergies (Patel and Greenberger 2019), immunological hyper-reactions (Ondari et al. 2021) or plain toxicoses as in St. Anthony's Fire (Al-Omari et al. 2018) increase the threat spectra for wide and diverse base biothreats outside the conventional host-symbiont/parasite injurious pattern.

Perhaps the best conceivable case of agents fully developed in their pathogenic status appearing *de novo*—and without any evolutionary warning, as is the case of pathogens evolving in historical times to more malign forms, like the multi-drug resistant Staphylococci (Howden et al. 2011)—refers to entities having evolved in total isolation or seclusion or behind some barrier. This is the case of exo-organisms (see Chapter 4), having evolved outside of the biosphere: on other celestial bodies or in enclaves once in contact with the rest of the biosphere and suddenly excluded and left to evolve independently for considerable time, due to some geologic or environmental event like earthquake, avalanche, ice-cap, etc. It should be kept in mind that evolutionary time is somewhat subjective. The release and ingress of such organisms may be the result of spontaneous events like climate change (discussed later) or the landing of meteorites, or exploration and exploitation routines like mining and deep-sea drilling; other drilling cases are also eligible for the list of risk factors, but to a lower extent. The ingress is expected to take place by both fomites and vectors. The former more so in the case of agents having been in stasis for long, as within glaciers; the latter in the case of isolated but fully functional enclaves, like caves sealed off by volcanic eruptions and earthquakes, without all the forms of life trapped within being purged by heat or poisonous gases.

The airstreams caused by different residual pressures in the enclave and out of it due to different etiologies (temperature change during the hours of the day is just an example), are the most usual means of translocation of the cryptic, isolated microbiomes. Water streams may function similarly, although the dispersion in this case could be slower. It may be detrimental to the marine organisms and this could have a tremendous impact on the entire planet. The colonization of land, where most of the humanomic expansion takes place, is more complicated; the microbes must survive the salt water (or freshwater for that matter) experience in terms of osmosis and predator microorganisms or viruses/phages, and then be resilient to non-aquatic environments to which they may be transferred by evaporation and rain, by periodic or circumstantial flooding of freshwater bodies such as lakes and rivers, by the tide or along the food chain and network. Boarding the equipment and the living agents of human-induced change such as mining would result in efficient and relatively long-range transportation and thus the initiation of more aggressive dissemination patterns.

In any case, the isolation would result in no specific immunity pathway (adaptive immunity) being co-developed causally to such potential pathogens (Xing et al. 2020), and without known antagonists, natural antimicrobials similar to antibiotics are less probable to come across; much less to come across promptly. Metabolomic analyses of whole new microbiomes may be required to discover analogues. The adaptive immunity mechanisms may be randomly applicable due to cross-reaction of paratopes with similar epitopes and to the inherently and purposely huge genetic instability of immunoglobulin genes (Pomés et al. 2020, Akbar et al. 2021). This could allow some optimism in that massive, extinction-level events may not be imminent; however, this applies to biological terms. It is well-understood that extinction may be caused much more probably as the result of a disruptive event rather than a destructive one: the damage and secondary casualties due to the measures taken and the failures of the social mechanics grossly outdid the actual death toll of COVID-19, which was not a very lethal virus (Zalla et al. 2022). Much of the said damage was due to the panic, less amidst commoners and more within authorities of different social prerogatives.

The above apply to different extents to xenoorganisms. The synthetic aspect of xenobiology, by definition, implies engineered organisms alien to the collective innate—and much more so to adaptive—immunity and to any communal system of countermeasures (see Chapter 4) such as natural antibiotics. Chance susceptibility may occasionally be expected (different probabilities apply to different batches and technologies of xenoorganisms), but, in principle, even diagnostic tests are expected to be ineffective. Xenoorganisms, developed occasionally to the exact specifications of legitimate end-users, are fully evolved and independently so from the biospheric microbiome, especially in adapted and restricted to their projected area of interest (target). The way such organisms may ingress the biosphere is, by definition, an issue of biosecurity. Perpetrated events are easy to guess as an issue, but from climate change events to true accidents, chance may have a saying, increasingly severe as the scale and popularity of the use of xenoorganisms increases.

Climate change affects the emergence of pathogens in multiple ways. Regarding the ones independently evolved and appearing full-fledged in terms of virulence factors, the causal link is the possibility that climate change caused events such as coastal or riverside floods and the thawing of ice, which may expose enclosed enclaves of cryptic microbiomes, independently evolving (exo-organisms) and introduce them into the wider biosphere, thus allowing their access to naïve host populations. The ones amongst such exo-organisms that have randomly acquired virulence factors applicable to the existing populations may have a disastrous free ride as the hosts are not prepared for their appearance and the adaptation by immunological pathways may prove ineffective in many cases. Consequently, it is conceivable that existential-level events may occur for species possibly essential for the ecosystem, but also for the network of dependence of human populations with the wild and the agrarian natural environments.

The geological history of the planet allows for the isolation of ecosystems in pockets due to geological events, such as earthquakes and volcanic eruptions, and conservation in stasis or through isolation by the formation of glaciers. The very fast onset of polar temperatures, resulting in mammoths being conserved in ice, with undigested plants in their stomachs and minimal if any necrotic degradation in tissues, presupposes similar speed in freezing microbiota, the physiology of which is much more resilient in deep-freezing, due to simplicity; as a result, thawing them may well bring them to fully active metabolic status, compatible with growth and propagation. The formation of hollows and enclaves maintained at viable temperatures due to volcanic and other heat sources within or under a ceiling of ice would conceivably produce ecosystems evolving similarly or dissimilarly to analogues in the biosphere and thus interchangeable in niche and prone to interaction. Events random in nature (such as earthquakes) or of human agency due to direct interventions (including urbanization, colonization and drilling/exploration), as mentioned earlier, may expose, dissolve and dilute such microbiomes into environmental liquids, including but not limited to the hydrosphere and the air, resulting in world-wide dispersion and a high probability of finding susceptible hosts.

2. Evolutionary emergence

This category directly and inescapably involves genomic factors and phenomena as it insinuates an existing agent that evolves to a pathogenic/virulent status within the same spatio-temporal continuum; meaning it is not transferred to another location, remote or otherwise naïve, nor is its presence intermittent. The new, malign strain coexists, at least temporarily, with the benign progenitor, but it may eventually surrogate the latter fully. The evolution may be spontaneous; when not spontaneous, it includes circumstances that accelerate evolution ('evolutionary factories' or 'incubators') and perpetrated/engineered pathways, which are discussed separately. The result is an agent with additional pathogenic functionality (gain-of-function) at the site where its benign ancestors had been thriving.

(i) Pressure by antibiotics

Evolution is promoted first and foremost by applying pressure to a population, and thus selecting evolved individuals instead of the ones following a previous, successful model. The abuse of antibiotics rapidly leads to the emergence of resistant strains; this happens faster than the formulation, testing and production of new compounds (Iskandar et al. 2022). The evolution of resistant strains is usually attributable to lateral gene transfer (LGT); *but* one should remember that the usual, vertical gene transfer (VGT) is focal in leading such traits to wide deployment within a population (Diwo and Budisa 2018). If the LGT causes lower propagation of the receiver, this could lead to a liability rather than an asset in evolutionary terms; the population may be exterminated by simple antagonism or by other challenges. Thus, the LGT *needs* an efficient, not disturbed, VGT to capitalize on the advantages it offers (Nagies et al. 2020); it is an evolutionary compromise to delete extreme characters, as is the classic issue of localized aggregation versus spatial dispersion encountered by many parasites of every kingdom of life (Nørgaard et al. 2019).

In this combination, one may detect a number of evolutionary dead ends regarding the development of resistant strains, or, in different terms, conclude that resistance development is much faster than observed. It is the combined effect of evolution and propagation efficiency that holds back the former's potential impact, which is a stern prediction, if it holds water, for perpetrated evolution and the gain-of-virulence by microorganisms.

The standard view of evolving microbial resistance to antimicrobial drugs at a rate that renders the latter obsolete and outpaces their development cycle (Iskandar et al. 2022) has two important afterthoughts. The first is regarding the existence a deterministic parameter as to how fast new compounds with antimicrobial characteristics are discovered or invented. When the pharmaceutical industry stops research on the subject because it is less profitable than other endeavors, the functional rate of developing antibiotics is expected to drop sharply; but this has nothing to do with technology, science or good practice or stewardship in the use of antibiotics. It is about failures in collective biosecurity strategy, which allow market considerations to take precedence over other ones, including scientific and social priorities (Kambouris et al. 2018a,b).

The second afterthought is that the same would be true for antiseptics, disinfectants and other microbicides or antimicrobials (Christensen and Brüggemann 2014, Nankervis et al. 2016) that were used indiscriminately and excessively during the COVID-19 pandemic as a hygiene *mantra* (Ghafoor et al. 2021). More potent in effect and less complicated in their *modus operandi* than the antibiotics, they are meant to tackle the pathogen before it enters the host, whence the fragile physiology of the latter allows no chemically or physically extreme measures to eradicate the invading or otherwise potentially harmful microbiota.

The use of such amenities is straightforward and so is the development of new ones: finding something that unsettles the physicochemical balance of a microbial cell without destroying organic and inorganic surrounding matter, mostly inanimate. This combination of characteristics—high destructiveness, wide applicability and no targeting/discrimination options—creates environmental havoc, deleting whole microbiomes indiscriminately whenever applied, thus affording rendering vacant habitats to transferred/transported or plainly drifting ones. Or—and this is worse—it deletes *parts* of microbiomes, allowing resilient taxa to flourish unobstructed and without ecological competition to reach such population numbers that create imbalance and aggressiveness, even if the cell physiology by itself is rather benign in normal conditions, when the population is checked by antagonistic subpopulations.

It is true that combined regimens might be a solution, as resistance is a condition that depletes the evolutionary potential of a microbe and it is difficult to co-evolve for resistance in more than one highly dissimilar threats, such as the combinations of antibiotics and antiseptics with physical amenities (heat, EM challenge-see Chapter 9) or biologicals (Caubet et al. 2004, Li et al. 2021). It is true that the elaborate interactions of antibiotics and resistance factors allowed, for some time, small but important changes to the chemical synthesis of antibiotics molecules (*modification*) to derail a very specific and elaborate targeted mechanism of resistance (Iskandar et al. 2022), occasionally endowing the molecule with better performance (*improvement*). This approach, however, has an expiration date: at some point of time, more generic, upstream resistance features will emerge and propagate, nullifying these shifts and the need will be in such cases to revert to highly divergent approaches.

In any case, the resistance in antibiotics does not create a pathogen, it increases the fitness of an existing one. A microbe does not cause disease because it is resistant to antibiotics; antibiotics are issued *after* disease is established and identified (to various degrees), except for the cases of prophylaxis (Segundo and Condino-Neto 2021). Even in the latter case, the microbe is not virulent because of its resistance; it may be because of its fast propagation, if nothing else, or due to some metabolite production, or due to selectivity or any other attribute, including its survivability against immune responses; but NOT due to its resistance against antibiotics.

As a result, it might have been a better idea to focus on denying gain of pathogenic/virulent function or to cause loss of functionality (pathogenicity/virulence actually) rather than spiraling into reactively treating disease with antibiotics and continually trying to develop better ones. Denying the physiological *and* micro-ecological elements of the gain-of-virulence, for instance when increasing the antagonism locally by administering biologicals (Bäumler and Sperandio 2016, Köhl et al. 2019), might be a more affordable, sustainable and perhaps even benign solution, as it does not delete entire microbiomes with one application.

(ii) Transportation-Travel-Migration (TTM)

The translocation of microbiota is important for functional emergence; in the realm of evolution though, even these events play a role, as the intense exchanges of matter and energy fuel evolution by sheer quantity of biomass amenable and subject to it. The availability of evolutionary substrate in traits and abundance of subjects is the second pillar of evolution. The TTM aspect of evolution reshapes microbiomes continuously, increases interface with humans and with the humanome, and brews adaptation pathways that may circumvent the host species barriers by randomness (open-loop) and also by reactive (closed-loop) evolution (Van Baarlen et al. 2007, Gillings 2017).

By the influx of new microbiota in volume due to transportation and translocation, new traits appear massively in established microbiomes, and the latter are reshuffled in two major ways: (a) by incorporating novel strains and taxa in general, as these are relocated, forming entirely new microbiomes, and (b) by incorporating new genomic elements into the genomes of the existing strains. Lateral gene transfer is a means to do so and such exchanges (which feedback the restructuring of the microbiomes, as mentioned above) are mostly performed through high-transmittance LGT options such as transduction, transposition and conjugation; transformation remains a valid option in high density populations, where cell debris is readily available and degradation of dead matter is slow and incomplete, creating a lot of e-DNA which is naked and partially decomposed, and hence easy to uptake (Neil et al. 2021). Thus, the evolution fed by TTM operates at both the levels of organism/population genetics and at the molecular level, by enriching the collective genome and the exogenome of a given location due to the influx of new strains.

The aspect of increased, massively populated microbiomes, occasionally diverse but in other cases disproportionately representing specific strains and/or higher taxa, is pivotal in the evolution of emerging pathogens. As mentioned above, the evolution may be prompted by pressure, or fueled by large populations in limited spatio-temporal settings, especially if there are subsets/subpopulations with novel traits which can be transferred as such or be subject to further genetic reshuffling and evolution. The TTM bring massive microbial loads from around the globe, endowed with peculiar traits, but in a haphazard way.

The same principle though is found to govern another, possibly more mischievous, line of events. High loads of microbiota are expected to operate in a targeted pattern and thus be less prone to dispersal. An exemplary such case is the use of selected strains as effectors of different processes, including but not limited to biomaturation of foodstuff, or as parts of different products, cheese products containing specific molds for instance. The industry of biomatured foodstuff (e.g., dairy products and wine) is the focus (Bouki et al. 2020), but many other cases should also be kept in mind. The advent of biopharmaceuticals/biologicals (Kesik-Brodacka 2018) and probiotics (Gasbarrini et al. 2016, *Probiotics: What You Need To Know* 2019) delivers, in a targeted fashion within prospective hosts, large populations of microbiota carrying massive DNA sequence loads that may join the collective exogenome and become available for LGT within the appendage microbiomes of the hosts.

(iii) High host population densities, faster evolution

The third pillar of the accelerated microbial evolution is the availability of hosts or habitats of plentiful nutrients and permissive conditions, where large populations of microbiota may grow, interact with high efficiency if mixed, and evolve if pure, at an increased pace due to non-deterministic (random) processes. In this category, one may see roughly two separate cases:

(a) Dense homogenous host populations which, even if not naïve, allow fast evolution by permitting successive and multiple infection cycles that, among other things, encourage recombination. This applies to both viruses that may infect the same host cells and thus recombine (Pérez-Losada et al. 2015), and conjugable prokaryota or even eukaryota (Danchin 2016) that coexist in limited volumes and may thus develop conjugation events at a higher pace than in less dense formats. High population density boroughs in megacities and concentration/refugee camps, especially in specific environments (humid) and those with substandard hygiene (which is the rule), come easily to mind in this context, and the explosively propagating populations of pests that act as vectors increase the interface and transmittance (MacFadden et al. 2018).

The intensive agricultural exploitation of breeding livestock—swine and poultry, as showcased in the swine and avian influenza epidemics (Walters 2014)—or the use of intensively cultivated, genetically homogenous plant strains in the great Irish famine (Goss et al. 2014) are much more important evolutionary risk factors than usually acknowledged. The threat for massive food production loss (Kambouris et al. 2018c) is only an obvious risk factor; insertion of virulent factors (mostly toxins) through the food chain (Miedaner and Geiger 2015) must never be underestimated, especially in the case of recombined ones, given the factors analyzed above. Also, it is regularly forgotten that many human pathogens are initially plant symbionts (Gauthier and Keller 2013) or much more often animal symbionts (Van Baarlen et al. 2007, Walker et al. 2018), that pass into the community through the interface of such species with humans. The transmission of plant or animal pathogens to human hosts through rats (Strand and Lundkvist 2019), migratory birds (Shah et al. 2022) or companion animals (Magouras et al. 2020) must not be overlooked. The expansion of the humanome in diverse and extended areas brings microbiota existing in secluded habitats, into interface and possible communion and recombination by allowing them to gain access to vast host populations with a large percentage of naïve prospective carriers, never previously exposed to such pathogens.

(b) The high volumes of biowaste allow a transient habitat to the newly introduced microbiota for them to settle, and from where they can jump to the new host species, with or without an evolution/adaptation step. Such cases include: (1) manure heaping in intensive breeding facilities (Gillings 2017, Bolan et al. 2021), (2) unspent quantities of organic/biological fertilizers, and discarded or uprooted green parts in plantations, including weeds, foliage and whole plants/trees/wood after the termination of a plantation (Aliaño-González et al. 2022), (3) the highly loaded urban sewage networks (Gillings 2017), and (4) eutrophication microbiomes (Paerl et al. 2003). Inoculated into massive quantities of biowaste, diverse microbiota may grow, with low selective pressure, to achieve high population density and thus achieve random evolution in their saprobiotic state. The intensive antagonism, even in the presence of and especially due to plentiful nutrients, may develop more aggressive strains spontaneously, which, if introduced into host environments (e.g., by contact, like through swimming in polluted recreational waters), would quickly outdo other strains (Vepštaitė-Monstavičė et al. 2018) long established in appendage microbiomes and thus, by becoming predominant by selection, reshape the said microbiomes to less balanced and more aggressive attitudes towards their hosts.

(iv) Combined evolutionary events and conditions

Under this title, occasions where the above pillars of evolution coexist may be presented. One such case is the indiscriminate use of probiotics as supplements, with little or no guidance concerning the diet and especially the drug intake. It is not that the said preparations massively introduce microbial populations that may rearrange even well-balanced appendage microbiomes or exert themselves pathogenicity, thus constituting a safety issue (Hanchi et al. 2018, Kothari et al. 2019); this is the obvious part. The problem that may arise is that in a nutrient-rich environment (human or animal or plant body), massive populations amenable to evolution are introduced, *plus* an agent that may accelerate or trigger evolution (such as prescription and non-prescription drugs and bioactive dietary habits that may exercise pressure on microbiomes), leading either to rearrangement by deleting susceptible—and not necessarily harmful—subpopulations (Ibragimova et al. 2021, Su and Liu 2021), or by creating possibly aggressive resistant strains (Hanchi et al. 2018, Kothari et al. 2019), or both! This is not limited to exposure to drugs and bioactive diet of probiotics (and, at a later stage, pharmabiotics, although the use of the latter is supposed to be better informed and monitored). Other environmental stimuli, such as the potent EM radiation (effected wherever 5G internet and cell phone (ab)use happens), are unappreciated as to their effect on spontaneous (meaning without evolutionary pressure exercised simultaneously) as well as prompted (adding pressure by a certified detrimental factor to the exposure to the basic stimulus) evolution of microbiota.

A similar issue is the biotech industry. It is expected to multiply its turnover in terms of use of biomass and of developing different lifeforms (Schmidt 2010), for it is considered a much more environmentally friendly and sustainable approach (Matthews et al. 2019), compared to gigantic synthetic industrial plants (Lokko et al. 2018, Candelon et al. 2022), greatly exceeding the turnovers of the more dispersed but lower-volume events described in (iii), which refer to small scale, end users rather than massive facilities. In the case of the latter, the concerned numbers are higher by several orders of magnitude, though their positional uncertainty is lower as they are expected to be found—and disperse from—major biotechnology facilities which are supposed to be registered and regulated (small, home breweries qualifying for inclusion in this category).

The engineered microorganisms may act as the source as well as the receivers of genomic elements that exist in other organisms or even freely in the environment (environmental DNA/e-DNA) the latter constitute the exogenome *sensu lato* (Kambouris et al. 2018a). Given that engineered microorganisms are expected to fulfill many different productive profiles (Wehrs et al. 2019, Osinubi et al. 2020) and that the industrial use ordinarily refers to the instrumentalization of extremely large populations of effector organisms, the evolutionary intensity is expected to be very high and just as unpredictable—a good reason for the discussion of a revamped xenobiological approach (Schmidt 2010). Additionally, the bioindustry is expected to multiply all the kinds of vectors as well: from engineered or bred organisms that may already be or later turn susceptible to microorganisms (García-Álvarez and Vallet-Regí 2022, Ratcliffe et al. 2022), to purposely manufactured vectors for delivery, in lab conditions or *in vivo* (as is the case with nucleic acid-based vaccines), of biochemical moieties (García-Álvarez and Vallet-Regí 2022) or executable genetic information (Mardanova et al. 2009, Brown et al. 2018, Scudellari 2019). The processes that are to occur once out of the regulated and controlled environment are expected to be massive; and, due to such massiveness, the predictability of detrimental outcomes is difficult to assess, but may be expected to be higher than the usual turnout by spontaneous evolution. The perpetrated or even the accidental aspects are not discussed herein, as they refer to events of a different pedigree, requiring more demanding measures of vigilance and resilience to discourage, deter, avert, contain and respond.

3. Functional emergence

This mechanism creates pathogens from existing non-pathogenic species, not by any gain-of-function and acquisition of virulence factors, but by changing the established routines, niches and balances amongst different microbiota and prospective or actual hosts.

(i) Climate change reshapes infectivity

It is easily understood that climate change may change the net infectivity of many microbial species. A warmer climate would decrease the thermal buffering afforded to warm-blooded animals by their increased inner (body) temperatures; microbiota evolved to optimally function at higher ambient temperatures would be less discouraged by such thermal buffering (Casadevall 2017, Sharma and Chakrabarti 2020). This is a well-understood prospect, and an obvious one. There are some additional spinoffs: whether the modified enzymes and the biochemical machinery of cells adapted to higher ambient temperatures would be as effective (or perhaps even more effective) against a number of challenges, including antimicrobial moieties. It is not as simple as it may seem: enzymes and other mechanisms (such as efflux channels) may work suboptimally in the said ambient temperatures, thus allowing more efficient protective microbicidal processes; or even quite the opposite (MacFadden et al. 2018) thus decon and antisepses rules may change. Given that the end phase of an infection will still be in a (human or other) host, such changes would not apply therapeutically or prophylactically, as the current microbial mechanisms seem perfectly functional, despite a more potent buffering. But this is only regarding humans and warm-blooded animals. Plants and cold-blooded animals are in another league altogether and therein, the interaction of the said enzymes and mechanisms of microbiota, attuned to the new environmental background, with existing antimicrobials/biocides (not limited to antibiotics) could well result in different efficiency patterns, for better or worse.

On the other hand, a higher ambient temperature means that low temperature would become a more formidable antimicrobial amenity, allowing better conservation of sensitive amenities such as medicinals and edibles. Whether psychrophilic conditions could become a norm for some exploitations is a valid question, especially in biotechnology. The possibility of freeze-shock, as against flame treatment, being used to promptly pasteurize equipment is undoubtedly intriguing and its practicality is to be assessed.

Environmental change is more complex than the mere rise of temperature. Humidity and wind are important for the dissemination and infectivity of microbiota that disperse through fomites; and the possibility of reservoirs of pathogens being introduced into the hydrosphere by the higher tides suggests by itself a reason for alarm, as immense populations of potentially pathogenic microorganisms would subsequently enter the planetary circulation through waters, waves and currents.

Humidity, on the other hand, allows better viability of xenobiota on the skin, one of its antimicrobial prerogatives being the semi-anhydrous environment which weakens microbiota and their ability to absorb and restore damage caused by antimicrobial peptides and other antimicrobial skin moieties (Schauber and Gallo 2008). Ambient moisture assists in extracellular hydrolytic reactions; the lysis of living or dead tissue which accompanies systemic infection, or local infection for that matter, is hydrolytic in nature (Navarro 2015). It also removes a limitation in the dispersion syllabus of a microbe—that is, the precaution of not being dehydrated and thus suffering desiccation (Pepper and Gerba 2015).

Different temperature and humidity would perhaps change the ambient chemical conditions, including the pH readings in many habitats. Before any new, evolved and adapted species emerge, it is certain that the existing microbiomes would be reshuffled, creating different combinations and habitats; these new microbiomes may be unstable, expansionist or outright aggressive towards existing and prospective hosts.

(ii) Immunodeficiency

Microorganisms of relatively low virulence show pathogenicity when accessing host populations of substandard immunity (Kärkkäinen et al. 2000, Ribes et al. 2000). This may refer to a partially derailed physiology due (a) to the standard of living, as in undernutrition or even malnutrition (Barazzoni et al. 2020), high density lodgings (MacFadden et al. 2018), which incidentally applies even more to agriculture, especially in intensive exploitations, and (b) to medical intervention. It has been a common suggestion, for many years, that medical and veterinary intervention with antibiotics increase the resistance of pathogenic microorganisms towards these amenities (Dyar et al. 2016; Kambouris et al. 2018a), as mentioned above in section (2) Evolutionary Emergence of this chapter. But the other side of the coin is that other interventions result in direct or indirect immunodeficiency—from the immunosuppression needed for transplantations (Roberts and Fishman 2021) and for regulating autoimmune syndromes (Sevim et al. 2019), to the immunodeficiency caused by aggressive antitumor treatment with radiological and chemical amenities (Aipire et al. 2020). The increase of life expectancy adds to the general population ages, by definition characterized by frailer immunities (Taylor and Raja 2022), resulting in mass casualties and evolutionary breweries. The former case has been well established in the case of the COVID-19 pandemic, wreaking havoc amongst senior citizens (Dhama et al. 2020). This was especially so in contexts of homogenous populations by age criteria, confined in close and limited spaces, as in seniors' lodgings, especially congested retirement homes, nursing homes and continuing care retirement communities (O'Driscoll et al. 2021).

The above prospects lead, in a best-case scenario, to the need of monitoring microbiomes (by regular screening), both the microenvironmental ones (as in places of work or residence), and the appendage ones, especially in highly vulnerable individuals (Wilson 2016). This is to issue prophylaxis, preferably without triggering new kinds and rounds of resistance development or reverse reactions.

Many conditions in the current everyday life lead to a relative degradation of immunity. These extend to very diverse categories—from lifestyle to accommodation, substandard air and water quality, heavy metal-corrupted diet and relatively high EM radiation due to the (ab)use of connectivity (El-Gohary and Said 2017). The possibility of expedited necrotic cell deaths may lead to vigorous cell proliferation which, under duress, may increase the rate of occurrence of neoplasmatic lesions (Collins et al. 1997). A higher rate of occurrence of such lesions burdens the immune system to reorient primarily to detecting and destroying tumors at an early stage, leaving less resources for combatting infections (Safdar et al. 2011). To this, it may be added that the use of antibiotics may have de-selected, in an evolutionary context, more robust and fit immune systems, as they did not constitute an evolutionary advantage within the contemporary human, animal or plant populations (Nitsch-Osuch 2017, Taylor and Raja 2022). This in turn means that now (and more so in the near future), even less fit pathogens or lower numbers of standard pathogens (meaning lower infectious doses) may establish themselves in numbers, positions and capacities causing infection, thus leading to higher numbers of incidents, enhanced pathogen dissemination, turnover and evolution and easier transmission of communicable diseases. It must be noted that although the stewardship of antibiotics is an established and proven good practice in human populations (Doron and Davidson 2011), it is, for many reasons, less widespread than expected (Dyar et al. 2016) and things are much worse with plant and animal populations of economic interest, which are selected for commercial characteristics and heavily drugged to avoid loss of yield and profit (Dyar et al. 2016, Kambouris et al. 2018c).

(iii) Microbiomic factors

(a) An important causative agent of infections are the appendage microbiomes, consisting of scores of potentially pathogenic strains, being deregulated (Bäumler and Sperandio 2016, Foster et al. 2017). The community—or the microorganism—which constitutes a localized microbiome is in balance with the macroorganism. Such a balance may not be what a microbe would call 'harmonious', as the populations are kept to relatively low numbers and in constant competition with one another (Foster et al. 2017); as a result, none may increase so as to become aggressive enough and threaten the physiology of the host, even to a local extent, by compromising the host's structure and function. Still, if this balance is off for any reason, either newcomers may establish themselves and thus reshape the microbiome, or the native populations may change their attitude.

In the former case, any microbiote from the environment, especially if aggressive or abundant enough ('enough' is of course a relative term), may colonize a biocompartment and flourish, especially if the said biocompartment is barren, e.g., due to the excessive use of antiseptics or any kind of decontaminant/

antimicrobial effector (see also Chapter 3), as before a major surgery (Sidhwa and Itani 2015), as well as prolonged antibiotic therapy (Rafii et al. 2008, Taylor and Raja 2022). In the absence of competition from other microbiota, the immigrant population may grow rapidly (Bäumler and Sperandio 2016). Additionally, the lack of other microflora due to microbiota depletion by any conceivable mechanism may have relaxed the residual antimicrobial factors of the system's innate immune response (Yang et al. 2021), thus allowing newcomers further room for growth. A vigorously growing population, by definition, will start producing detrimental effects and thus cause an inflammation and perhaps an infection (Willems et al. 2020), which may remain localized or breach the skin barrier, invade and disperse, or even transit by autoinfection to other, more susceptible and vulnerable body parts/biocompartments. Thus, the elimination of the resident, native flora may turn a migrating agent into a pathogen due to permissive conditions (Bäumler and Sperandio 2016).

Similarly, in the latter case, the deregulation of the appendage microbiome due to the deletion or degradation of one or more strains' populations and/or a change in the biochemical environment may benefit some native (not migrating), potentially pathogenic, species/strain. On one hand, if the staphylococci are taken as an example, drug-resistant strains, if naturally occurring, are less fit towards other environmental and ecological challenges (Lowy 2003, Vogwill and MacLean 2015) and, as a result, backrunners in fitness contests. The removal of antagonistic populations potentially results in less exposure to microbial antimicrobials and more available nutrients. On the other hand, beneficial changes in environmental factors may include (i) different pH, as the human skin is usually at a slightly acidic pH which is restrictive for many mesophilic microbiota (Kurabayashi et al. 2002, Ali and Yosipovitch 2013), (ii) diminished release of antimicrobial peptides and antibodies (Schauber and Gallo 2008), and (iii) increase of secretions better suited to the metabolic needs and the physiological mechanism of a given microbiote. As a result, handicapped but virulent (possibly but not necessarily drug-resistant) strains may be promoted in the fitness race against their peers, grow fast and extensively, and ultimately cause disease.

(b) The use of live microorganisms as a pharmaceutical treatment, under the guise of biopharmaceuticals and pharmabiotics, would increase the ingestion of microbiota manifold, compared to probiotics (Kothari et al. 2019) and perhaps rough/unpasteurized foodstuff and beverages, especially in the highly urbanized, medium to low income social strata. The mechanism of such populations, some of them by definition liable to become pathogenic, such as the enterococci (Hanchi et al. 2018, Krawczyk et al. 2021), is similar to the ones described above. Given the massiveness of the gastrointestinal tract (GIT) microbiome, or of other microbiomes in other prospective applications, deregulation could well be as probable as regulation, especially under duress and unstable diet and everyday routine (sleep routine, prescription or off-the-self drug intake, smoking and alcohol consumption). As a result, populations may become overabundant and cause septic/infectious events, although this would be, even in an epidemic, epidemiologically limited and geographically restricted by the non-contagious nature of the event. On the other hand, the toxicosis due to such agents is a much more probable cause for concern, and poor marketing or manufacturing practices could lead to massive outbreaks due to a common denominator rather than a serial expansion of cases. Foul play in any step of production and supply chain(s) would never be out of the question, turning a basically biosafety issue into a biosecurity nightmare. The migration of such populations to other biocompartments is a valid reason for additional concern; vomiting may allow colonization of the nasal cavity, the respiratory tract and sinuses, by the GIT microbiome, and this is but one example. The reduced resilience of the respiratory tract towards infectious agents, compared to the very hostile and acidic environment of the GIT, would imply that even benign microbiota of the GIT microbiome could be reasons for concern, and if proprietary/engineered strains are used, such concerns may understandably grow. Without even taking into consideration the LGT dimension, the use (prescribed or otherwise) of live microorganisms should be closely monitored and regulated (Kothari et al. 2019).

(iv) Translocation

Massive amounts of microbiota and eventually whole microbiomes move around the globe on a daily basis (Nitsch-Osuch 2017, Grobusch et al. 2020). Although endemism is a standard prerogative for microbes and microbiomes (Choudoir et al. 2018, Richter-Heitmann et al. 2020) intercontinental distances are covered within a day in some cases, while in other cases, intercontinental treks taking months to complete create a stream of microbial exchange and amplify emigrant cells to immigrant populations. The main mechanisms for such translocation are Transportation, Travel and Migration (TTM) as mentioned above in this chapter. Migration applies to both the cases mentioned above, while Travel usually applies to the former case, i.e., prompt translocation, and Transportation, especially regarding trade, mostly to the latter, slow and massive translocation, occurring due to the sheer volume of produce changing hands and markets. Transplanted, or rather translocated microbiota find themselves in new geographical, environmental and microbiological conditions and may adopt traits different from the source populations in the original habitat(s). The usual example is the transmittable diseases that decimated, to different degrees, the populations of both the Old and the New Worlds as the respective agents found naïve host populations (i.e., permissive microbiological conditions) to propagate in; for instance, smallpox effectively destroyed the native populations in South and Central America (Patterson and Runge 2002, Thèves et al. 2016, Kambouris 2021b). Permissive environmental conditions, coupled with favorable ecological/microbiological ones, turned a serious plant pathogen, *Phytophthora infestans*, into a mass murderer—a GCBR in modern parlance—by providing excellent dissemination conditions throughout a dense and naïve host population (Goss et al. 2014, Kambouris 2021b). Geography is always a concern, as it may also affect bioagents, in terms of weather, macroclimate, photoperiod and endemism, along with the seasonal variance of microbiomes (Choudoir et al. 2018, Richter-Heitmann et al. 2020). And this does not apply only to microorganisms; macroorganisms (e.g., insects) constitute a very real part of the translocatable threat, either as vectors or as effectors/natural enemies.

The vector mosquito of malaria, *Anopheles*, is an example of the former (Prabhu et al. 2022) and *Phylloxera* of the latter (Tello et al. 2019). Although the risk usually remains endemic rather than epidemic, at least in spontaneous outbreaks, indirect intercontinental translocation of insects has also been detected, e.g., *Lycorma delicatula*, a very invasive and destructive species regarding soybean, orchard trees and other plants, that originated in China but currently spread and plights the US (*USDA* n. d.).

The volume of travelers and the density of travel and transportation patterns create major risks for massive delivery/ingress of highly transmittable microbiota and pests (Ratcliffe et al. 2022), especially if the latter are characterized by short incubation times. Poor hygiene along with physical deterioration and low groundspeed make the immigrant routes high-risk factors for pathogens transmitted through fomites and secondary vectors/carriers (Khalil and Shinwari 2015, Tuite et al. 2018), while the trade of live and dead organic matter (e.g., timber and crops) transports masses of opportunistic pathogens, possibly toxin-producing ones with an eminent saprophytic phase, e.g., aphlatoxin-producing *Aspergillus flavus* (Mitema 2019, Yang et al. 2020).

The manifestation of increased, unexpected aggressiveness and the consequent impact by a newly translocated microbe, regardless of any previous congenital pathogenic activity, may need some time to occur, so as to adapt to the new conditions and hosts; sometimes though, this might not be so. The latter is the case when the microenvironement is very similar, although the host and the macroenvironment may vary considerably. For example, similar vaginal biochemistry would favor *Candida* infections throughout very different human populations, or even other species (Cleff et al. 2005, Willems et al. 2020).

The above is a textbook case; the integrative dimension is potentially more intriguing. In many cases, it is not just individual pathogens or pathogen populations, meaning a single species/strain, but entire microbiomes that are translocated; e.g., a piece of a biofilm on a trunk which is loaded and transported as timber. The translocation of these microbiomes, which is most common when addressing massive, poorly sanitized influx of matter (e.g., trade), could be pivotal in the possible emergence of a pathogen. For example, a chaperone organism, the best example being helper/satellite virus complexes (Hu et al. 2009), may be instrumental for a pathogen's infectious cycle, and this helper species/strain may be more susceptible to a change in habitat. Consequently, the translocated microbiomes could brew biosecurity issues unpredictable by the mere listing the microbiota they include.

The massive nature of such translocation, with billions or trillions of cells moved daily to new environments, means a higher degree of contact of the translocated microbes with humans and the humanome in general, both during the process (as in migration) and as its end result (as in trade). The contact of massive amounts of microbiota with new populations allows more opportunities for the evolution of aggressive strains as a result of the said interface and interaction simply due to statistics. Higher numbers of cells, given the opportunity to colonize new hosts, imply more possibilities for successful adaptation to these hosts, translatable to even more individuals that are to eventually disperse to more loci where interface occurs. It also implies a higher rate of new characters being created and tried by natural selection, compared to if such contacts were kept minimum. Less interface implies less possibilities for finding susceptible hosts presenting immune defects or especially compliant adhesion characters, and thus less opportunities for entering a new host whence the pathogen may evolve or disseminate as is. By sensibly pasteurizing or at least sanitizing or decontaminating loads of merchandize and people, a process hitherto unimaginable, but now less so due to COVID-19 (Grobusch et al. 2020), this mass production of new, evolved and adapted pathogens from benign microbiomes may be curtailed dramatically. In the case of COVID-19, such measures were meant to stop transmission (Sharma et al. 2021), but from a more generic and advanced perspective, the objective is to avoid not the direct *infections* caused due to the transmission of ready-made killer pathogens, but the *evolution* of such pathogens due to the transmission of massive population loads of benign or conventional microbiota that may evolve to the status of superbug/superpathogen or neopathogen (Kambouris 2021a).

References

Aipire, A. et al. (2020). The immunostimulatory activity of polysaccharides from Glycyrrhiza uralensis. PeerJ, 8(1). doi: 10.7717/PEERJ.8294.

Akbar, R. et al. (2021). A compact vocabulary of paratope-epitope interactions enables predictability of antibody-antigen binding. Cell Reports, 34(11): 108856. doi: 10.1016/J.CELREP.2021.108856.

Al-Omari, R. et al. (2018). Clinical uses and toxicity of Ergot, Claviceps purpurea An evidence-based comprehensive retrospective review (2003–2017). Bioscience Biotechnology Research Communications, 11(3): 356–362. doi: 10.21786/BBRC/11.3/2.

Ali, S.M. and Yosipovitch, G. (2013). Skin pH: From basic science to basic skin care. Acta Dermato-Venereologica, 93(3): 261–267. doi: 10.2340/00015555-1531/.

Aliaño-González, M.J. et al. (2022). Wood waste from fruit trees: Biomolecules and their applications in agri-food industry. Biomolecules, 12(2): 238. doi: 10.3390/BIOM12020238.

Van Baarlen, P. et al. (2007). Molecular mechanisms of pathogenicity: How do pathogenic microorganisms develop cross-kingdom host jumps? FEMS Microbiology Reviews, 31(3): 239–277. doi: 10.1111/J.1574-6976.2007.00065.X.

Barazzoni, R. et al. (2020). ESPEN expert statements and practical guidance for nutritional management of individuals with SARS-CoV-2 infection. Clinical Nutrition, 39(6): 1631–1638. doi: 10.1016/J.CLNU.2020.03.022.

Batista, B.G. et al. (2020). Human fusariosis: An emerging infection that is difficult to treat. Revista da Sociedade Brasileira de Medicina Tropical, 53: 1–7. doi: 10.1590/0037-8682-0013-2020.

Bäumler, A.J. and Sperandio, V. (2016). Interactions between the microbiota and pathogenic bacteria in the gut. Nature, 535(7610): 85–93. doi: 10.1038/nature18849.

Begg, K.J. and Donachie, W.D. (1998). Division planes alternate in spherical cells of *Escherichia coli*. Journal of Bacteriology, 180(9): 2564–2567. doi: 10.1128/JB.180.9.2564-2567.1998.

Bolan, N. et al. (2021). Distribution, behaviour, bioavailability and remediation of poly- and per-fluoroalkyl substances (PFAS) in solid biowastes and biowaste-treated soil. Environment International, 155: 106600. doi: 10.1016/J.ENVINT.2021.106600.

Bonner, J.T. (2004). Perspective: The size-complexity rule. Evolution; International Journal of Organic Evolution, 58(9): 1883–1890. doi: 10.1111/J.0014-3820.2004.TB00476.X.

Bordenstein, S.R. and Theis, K.R. (2015). Host biology in light of the microbiome: Ten principles of holobionts and hologenomes. PLoS Biology, 13(8). doi: 10.1371/JOURNAL.PBIO.1002226.

Bouki, P. et al. (2020). Microbiomic prospects in fermented food and beverage technology. pp. 245–277. *In*: Kambouris, M.E. and Velegraki, A. (eds.). Microbiomics: Dimensions, Applications, and Translational Implications of Human and Environmental Microbiome Research. Elsevier. doi: 10.1016/B978-0-12-816664-2.00012-8.

Brown, H.C. et al. (2018). Target-cell-directed bioengineering approaches for gene therapy of hemophilia A', Molecular Therapy. Methods & Clinical Development. American Society of Gene & Cell Therapy, 9: 57. doi: 10.1016/J.OMTM.2018.01.004.

Canale-Parola, E. and Wolfe, R.S. (1960). Studies on Sarcina ventriculi. Journal of Bacteriology, 79(6): 857–62. doi: 10.1128/jb.79.6.857-859.1960.

Candelon, F. et al. (2022). Synthetic Biology Is About to Disrupt Your Industry, Global management consulting publications. Available at: https://www.bcg.com/publications/2022/synthetic-biology-is-about-to-disrupt-your-industry (Accessed: 23 April 2022).

Casadevall, A. (2017). Don't forget the fungi when considering global catastrophic biorisks. Health Security, 15(4): 341–342. doi: 10.1089/hs.2017.0048.

Caubet, R. et al. (2004). A radio frequency electric current enhances antibiotic efficacy against bacterial biofilms. Antimicrobial Agents and Chemotherapy, 48(12): 4662–4664. doi: 10.1128/AAC.48.12.4662-4664.2004.

Choudoir, M.J. et al. (2018). Variation in range size and dispersal capabilities of microbial taxa. Ecology, 99(2): 322–334. doi: 10.1002/ECY.2094.

Christensen, G.J.M. and Brüggemann, H. (2014). Bacterial skin commensals and their role as host guardians. Beneficial Microbes, 5(2): 201–215. doi: 10.3920/BM2012.0062.

Cieslak, T.J. et al. (2018). Beyond the dirty dozen: a proposed methodology for assessing future bioweapon threats. Military Medicine, 183(1-2): e59–e65. doi: 10.1093/MILMED/USX004.

Cleff, M.B. et al. (2005). Isolation of *Candida* spp. from vaginal microbiota of healthy canine females during estrous cycle. Brazilian Journal of Microbiology, 36(2): 201–204. doi: 10.1590/S1517-83822005000200018.

Cleland, C.E. and Copley, S.D. (2005). The possibility of alternative microbial life on Earth. International Journal of Astrobiology, 4(3-4): 165–173. doi: 10.1017/S147355040500279X.

Colf, L.A. (2016). Preparing for nontraditional biothreats. Health Security, 14(1): 7–12. doi: 10.1089/HS.2015.0045.

Collins, K. et al. (1997). The cell cycle and cancer. Proceedings of the National Academy of Sciences of the United States of America, 94(7): 2776–2778. doi: 10.1073/PNAS.94.7.2776.

Dance, A. (2021). The shifting sands of "gain-of-function" research. Nature, 598(7882): 554–557. doi: 10.1038/D41586-021-02903-X.

Danchin, E.G.J. (2016). Lateral gene transfer in eukaryotes: Tip of the iceberg or of the ice cube. BMC Biology, 14(1): 1–3. doi: 10.1186/S12915-016-0330-X/FIGURES/1.

Devos, D.P. et al. (2014). Evolution of the nucleus. Current Opinion in Cell Biology. Curr Opin Cell Biol, 28(100): 8–15. doi: 10.1016/J.CEB.2014.01.004.

Dhama, K. et al. (2020). COVID-19 in the elderly people and advances in vaccination approaches.Human Vaccines & Immunotherapeutics, 16(12): 2938–2943. doi: 10.1080/21645515.2020.1842683.

diCenzo, G.C. and Finan, T.M. 2017. The divided bacterial genome: Structure, function, and evolution. Microbiol Mol Biol Rev, 81:e00019-17. https://doi.org/10.1128/MMBR.00019-17.

Diwo, C. and Budisa, N. (2018). Alternative biochemistries for alien life: Basic concepts and requirements for the design of a robust biocontainment system in genetic isolation. Genes, 10(1). doi: 10.3390/genes10010017.

Doron, S. and Davidson, L.E. (2011). Antimicrobial stewardship. Mayo Clinic Proceedings, 86(11): 1113–1123. doi: 10.4065/mcp.2011.0358.

Dyar, O.J. et al. (2016). Using antibiotics responsibly: Are we there yet? Future Microbiology, 11(8): 1057–1071. doi: 10.2217/fmb-2016-0041.

El-Gohary, O.A. and Said, M.A.A. (2017). Effect of electromagnetic waves from mobile phone on immune status of male rats: Possible protective role of vitamin D. Canadian Journal of Physiology and Pharmacology, 95(2): 151–156. doi: 10.1139/CJPP-2016-0218.

Foster, K.R. et al. (2017). The evolution of the host microbiome as an ecosystem on a leash. Nature, 548(7665): 43–51.

García-Álvarez, R. and Vallet-Regí, M. (2022). Bacteria and cells as alternative nano-carriers for biomedical applications. Expert Opin Drug Deliv, 19(1): 103–118. doi: 10.1080/17425247.2022.2029844.

Gasbarrini, G. et al. (2016). Probiotics History. Journal of Clinical Gastroenterology, 50: S116–S119. doi: 10.1097/MCG.0000000000000697.

Gauthier, G.M. and Keller, N.P. (2013). Crossover fungal pathogens: The biology and pathogenesis of fungi capable of crossing kingdoms to infect plants and humans. Fungal Genetics and Biology, 61: 146–157. doi: 10.1016/J.FGB.2013.08.016.

Ghafoor, D. et al. (2021). Excessive use of disinfectants against COVID-19 posing a potential threat to living beings. Current Research in Toxicology, 2: 159–168. doi: 10.1016/J.CRTOX.2021.02.008.

Ghoul, M. and Mitri, S. (2016). Special series: microbial communities the ecology and evolution of microbial competition. Trends in Microbiology, 24: 833–845. doi: 10.1016/j.tim.2016.06.011.

Gillings, M.R. (2017). Lateral gene transfer, bacterial genome evolution, and the Anthropocene. Ann N Y Acad Sci, 1389(1): 20–36. doi: 10.1111/nyas.13213.

Goss, E.M. et al. (2014). The Irish potato famine pathogen Phytophthora infestans originated in central Mexico rather than the Andes. Proceedings of the National Academy of Sciences, 111(24): 8791–8796. doi: 10.1073/pnas.1401884111.

Grobusch, M.P. et al. (2020). Air travel and COVID-19 prevention: Fasten your seat belts, turbulence ahead. Travel Medicine and Infectious Disease, 38: 101927. doi: 10.1016/J.TMAID.2020.101927.

Hanchi, H. et al. (2018). The genus Enterococcus: Between probiotic potential and safety concerns-an update. Frontiers in Microbiology, 9: 1791. doi: 10.3389/FMICB.2018.01791/BIBTEX.

Hendrickson, H.L. and Poole, A.M. (2018). Manifold Routes to a Nucleus. Frontiers in Microbiology, 9: 2604. doi: 10.3389/FMICB.2018.02604.

Hibbing, M.E. et al. (2010). Bacterial competition: Surviving and thriving in the microbial jungle. Nature reviews. Microbiology, 8(1): 15. doi: 10.1038/NRMICRO2259.

Homeland Security Presidential Directive/HSPD-18-Medical Countermeasures Against Weapons of Mass Destruction (2007).

Howden, B.P. et al. (2011). Evolution of multidrug resistance during *Staphylococcus aureus* infection involves mutation of the essential two component regulator WalKR. PLoS pathogens, 7(11): e1002359. doi: 10.1371/JOURNAL.PPAT.1002359.

Hu, C.C. et al. (2009). Satellite RNAs and satellite viruses of plants. Viruses, 1(3): 1325–1350. doi: 10.3390/V1031325.

Ibragimova, S. et al. (2021). Dietary patterns and associated microbiome changes that promote oncogenesis. Frontiers in Cell and Developmental Biology, 9: 3210. doi: 10.3389/FCELL.2021.725821/BIBTEX.

Iskandar, K. et al. (2022). Antibiotic discovery and resistance: the chase and the race. Antibiotics, 11(2): 182. doi: 10.3390/ANTIBIOTICS11020182.

Kambouris, M. (2021a). Bio-offense: Black biology. pp. 109–126. *In*: Kambouris, M. (ed.). Genomics in Biosecurity. 1st edn. London: Elsevier Academic Press.

Kambouris, M. (2021b). Global catastrophic biological risks: Nature and response. pp. 29–42. *In*: Kambouris, M.E. (ed.). Genomics in Biosecurity. 1st edn. London: Elsevier Academic Press.

Kambouris, M.E. et al. (2018a). Humanome versus microbiome: Games of dominance and pan-biosurveillance in the Omics Universe. OMICS A Journal of Integrative Biology, 22(8): 528–538. doi: 10.1089/omi.2018.0096.

Kambouris, M.E. et al. (2018b). Rebooting bioresilience: A multi-OMICS approach to tackle global catastrophic biological risks and next-generation biothreats. OMICS A Journal of Integrative Biology, 22(1): 35–51. doi: 10.1089/omi.2017.0185.

Kambouris, M.E. et al. (2018c). Toward decentralized agrigenomic surveillance? A polymerase chain reaction-restriction fragment length polymorphism approach for adaptable and rapid detection of user-defined fungal pathogens in potato crops. OMICS A Journal of Integrative Biology, 22(4): 264–73. doi: 10.1089/omi.2018.0012.

Kambouris, M. and Velegraki, A. (2020). Introduction: The microbiome as a concept: Vogue or necessity? pp. 1–4. *In*: Kambouris, M.E. and Velegraki, A. (eds.). Microbiomics: Dimensions, Applications, and Translational Implications of Human and Environmental Microbiome Research. 1st edn. Elsevier Academic Press.

Kambouris, M.E. et al. (2022). Beyond the microbiome: Germ-ganism? An Integrative Idea for Microbial Existence, Organization, Growth, Pathogenicity, and Therapeutics. Omics : A Journal of Integrative Biology, 26(4): 204–217. doi: 10.1089/OMI.2022.0015.

Kärkkäinen, U.M. et al. (2000). Low virulence of *Escherichia coli* strains causing urinary tract infection in renal disease patients. European Journal of Clinical Microbiology & Infectious Diseases, 19(4): 254–259. doi: 10.1007/S100960050472.

Kesik-Brodacka, M. (2018). Progress in biopharmaceutical development. Biotechnology and Applied Biochemistry, 65(3): 306. doi: 10.1002/BAB.1617.

Khalil, A.T. and Shinwari, Z.K. (2015). Threats of agricultural bioterrorism to an agro dependent economy; What should be done? Journal of Bioterrorism & Biodefense, 05(01): 1–8. doi: 10.4172/2157-2526.1000127.

Köhl, J. et al. (2019). Mode of action of microbial biological control agents against plant diseases: Relevance beyond efficacy. Frontiers in Plant Science, 10: 845. doi: 10.3389/FPLS.2019.00845/BIBTEX.

Kothari, D. et al. (2019). Probiotic supplements might not be universally-effective and safe: A review. Biomedicine & Pharmacotherapy, 111: 537–547. doi: 10.1016/J.BIOPHA.2018.12.104.

Krawczyk, B. et al. (2021). The many faces of *Enterococcus* spp.—Commensal, Probiotic and Opportunistic Pathogen. Microorganisms, 9(9): 1900. doi: 10.3390/MICROORGANISMS9091900.

Kurabayashi, H. et al. (2002). Inhibiting bacteria and skin pH in hemiplegia: effects of washing hands with acidic mineral water. American Journal of Physical Medicine & Rehabilitation, 81(1): 40–46. doi: 10.1097/00002060-200201000-00007.

Laurence, M. (2020). Metagenomics in Microbiomic Studies. pp. 121–155. *In:* Kambouris, M. and Velegraki, A. (eds.). Microbiomics: Dimensions, Applications, and Translational Implications of Human and Environmental Microbiome Research. ELSEVIER ACADEMIC PRESS.

Li, X. et al. (2021). A combination therapy of Phages and Antibiotics: Two is better than one. International Journal of Biological Sciences, 17(13): 3573. doi: 10.7150/IJBS.60551.

Lokko, Y. et al. (2018). Biotechnology and the bioeconomy—Towards inclusive and sustainable industrial development. New Biotechnology, 40: 5–10. doi: 10.1016/J.NBT.2017.06.005.

Lovgren, S. (2003). HIV Originated With Monkeys, Not Chimps, Study Finds, National Geographic. Available at: https://www.nationalgeographic.com/science/article/news-hiv-aids-monkeys-chimps-origin (Accessed: 19 April 2022).

Lowy, F.D. (2003). Antimicrobial resistance: the example of Staphylococcus aureus. Journal of Clinical Investigation, 111(9): 1265. doi: 10.1172/JCI18535.

MacFadden, D.R. et al. (2018). Antibiotic resistance increases with local temperature. Nature Climate Change, 8(6): 510–514. doi: 10.1038/s41558-018-0161-6.

Magouras, I. et al. (2020). Emerging zoonotic diseases: should we rethink the animal–human interface? Frontiers in Veterinary Science, 7: 582743. doi: 10.3389/FVETS.2020.582743/BIBTEX.

Mardanova, E.S. et al. (2009). The optimization of viral vector translation improves the production of recombinant proteins in plants. Molecular Biology, 43(3): 524–527. doi: 10.1134/S0026893309030212.

Márquez-Zacarías, P. et al. (2021). Why have aggregative multicellular organisms stayed simple? Current Genetics, 67(6): 871–876. doi: 10.1007/S00294-021-01193-0.

Matthews, N.E. et al. (2019). Collaborating constructively for sustainable biotechnology. Scientific Reports, 9(1): 1–15. doi: 10.1038/s41598-019-54331-7.

Miedaner, T. and Geiger, H.H. (2015). Biology, genetics, and management of ergot (*Claviceps* spp.) in rye, sorghum, and pearl millet. Toxins. 7(3): 659–678. doi: 10.3390/toxins7030659.

Mitema, A. et al. (2019). The development of a qPCR assay to measure *Aspergillus flavus* biomass in maize and the use of a biocontrol strategy to limit aflatoxin production. Toxins. Basel, 11(3). doi: 10.3390/TOXINS11030179.

Nagies, F.S.P. et al. (2020). A spectrum of verticality across genes. PLOS Genetics, 16(11): e1009200. doi: 10.1371/JOURNAL.PGEN.1009200.

Nankervis, H. et al. (eds.) (2016). Antimicrobials including antibiotics, antiseptics and antifungal agents. *In*: Scoping systematic review of treatments for eczema. Southampton: NIHR Journals Library.

Navarro, M. (2015). Destructins and the Hydrolytic Power of a Fungal Infection. Ask batman. Available at: https://www.linkedin.com/pulse/destructins-hydrolytic-power-fungal-infection-ask-batman-navarro (Accessed: 21 April 2022).

Neil, K. et al. (2021). Molecular mechanisms influencing bacterial conjugation in the intestinal microbiota. Frontiers in Microbiology, 12: 1415. doi: 10.3389/FMICB.2021.673260/BIBTEX.

Nitsch-Osuch, A. (2017) '[Travels and spreading of multi-resistant bacteria]', Polski merkuriusz lekarski : organ Polskiego Towarzystwa Lekarskiego, 42(251): 219–222.

Nørgaard, L.S. et al. (2019). Can pathogens optimize both transmission and dispersal by exploiting sexual dimorphism in their hosts? Biology Letters, 15(6). doi: 10.1098/RSBL.2019.0180.

O'Driscoll, M. et al. (2021). Age-specific mortality and immunity patterns of SARS-CoV-2. Nature, 590(7844): 140–145. doi: 10.1038/S41586-020-2918-0.

Ondari, E. et al. (2021). Eosinophils and Bacteria, the Beginning of a Story. International Journal of Molecular Sciences, 22(15). doi: 10.3390/IJMS22158004.

Osinubi, K.J. et al. (2020). Review of the use of microorganisms in geotechnical engineering applications. SN Applied Sciences, 2(2): 1–19. doi: 10.1007/S42452-020-1974-2.

Özdemir, V. (2018). The dark side of the moon: the internet of things, industry 4.0, and the quantified Planet. OMICS: A Journal of Integrative Biology, 22(10): 637–641. doi: 10.1089/omi.2018.0143.

Paerl, H.W. et al. (2003). Microbial indicators of aquatic ecosystem change: Current applications to eutrophication studies. FEMS Microbiology Ecology, 46(3): 233–246. doi: 10.1016/S0168-6496(03)00200-9.

Paolillo, C. et al. (2019). Single-cell genomics. Clinical Chemistry, 65(8): 972–985. doi: 10.1373/CLINCHEM.2017.283895.

Patel, G. and Greenberger, P.A. (2019). Allergic bronchopulmonary aspergillosis. Allergy and Asthma Proceedings, 40(6): 421–424. doi: 10.2500/AAP.2019.40.4262.

Patterson, K.B. and Runge, T. (2002). Smallpox and the Native American. American Journal of the Medical Sciences, 323(4): 216–222. doi: 10.1097/00000441-200204000-00009.

Pepper, I.L. and Gerba, C.P. (2015). Aeromicrobiology. In: Pepper, I.L. et al. (eds.). Environmental Microbiology. Elsevier, p. 89. doi: 10.1016/B978-0-12-394626-3.00005-3.

Pérez-Losada, M. et al. (2015). Recombination in viruses: Mechanisms, methods of study, and evolutionary consequences. Infection, Genetics and Evolution, 30: 296. doi: 10.1016/J.MEEGID.2014.12.022.

Perry, M. (2019). 50 years of failed doomsday, eco-pocalyptic predictions; the so-called 'experts' are 0-50. American Enterprise Institute. Available at: https://www.aei.org/carpe-diem/50-years-of-failed-doomsday-eco-pocalyptic-predictions-the-so-called-experts-are-0-50/ (Accessed: 23 April 2022).

Pomés, A. et al. (2020). Structural aspects of the allergen-antibody interaction.Frontiers in Immunology, 11: 2067. doi: 10.3389/FIMMU.2020.02067/BIBTEX.

Prabhu, S.R. et al. (2022). Malaria epidemiology and COVID-19 pandemic: are they interrelated? Omics : A Journal of Integrative Biology, 26(4): 179–188. doi: 10.1089/OMI.2021.0227.

Probiotics: What You Need To Know (2019) NCCIH. Available at: https://www.nccih.nih.gov/health/probiotics-what-you-need-to-know (Accessed: 23 April 2022).

Rafii, F. et al. (2008). Effects of treatment with antimicrobial agents on the human colonic microflora. Therapeutics and Clinical Risk Management, 4(6): 1343. doi: 10.2147/TCRM.S4328.

Ratcliffe, N.A. et al. (2022). Overview of paratransgenesis as a strategy to control pathogen transmission by insect vectors. Parasites & Vectors, 15(1): 1–31. doi: 10.1186/S13071-021-05132-3.

Ribes, J.A. et al. (2000). Zygomycetes in human disease. Clinical Microbiology Reviews, 13(2): 236–301. doi: 10.1128/CMR.13.2.236.

Richter-Heitmann, T. et al. (2020). stochastic dispersal rather than deterministic selection explains the spatio-temporal distribution of soil bacteria in a temperate grassland. Frontiers in Microbiology, 11: 1391. doi: 10.3389/FMICB.2020.01391/BIBTEX.

Roberts, M.B. and Fishman, J.A. (2021). Immunosuppressive agents and infectious risk in transplantation: Managing the "Net State of Immunosuppression". Clinical Infectious Diseases, 73(7): e1302–e1317. doi: 10.1093/CID/CIAA1189.

Safdar, A. et al. (2011). Infections in patients with cancer: overview. Principles and Practice of Cancer Infectious Diseases, 2011: 3–15. doi: 10.1007/978-1-60761-644-3_1.

Schauber, J. and Gallo, R.L. (2008). Antimicrobial peptides and the skin immune defense system. The Journal of Allergy and Clinical Immunology, 122(2): 261. doi: 10.1016/J.JACI.2008.03.027.

Schmidt, M. (2010). Xenobiology: A new form of life as the ultimate biosafety tool. BioEssays, 32(4): 322–331. doi: 10.1002/bies.200900147.

Scudellari, M. (2019). Self-destructing mosquitoes and sterilized rodents: The promise of gene drives. Nature Research, 571(7764): 160–162. doi: 10.1038/D41586-019-02087-5.

Segundo, G.R.S. and Condino-Neto, A. (2021). Treatment of patients with immunodeficiency: Medication, gene therapy, and transplantation. Jornal de Pediatria, 97: S17–S23. doi: 10.1016/J. JPED.2020.10.005.

Sevim, E. et al. (2019). Is there a role for immunosuppression in antiphospholipid syndrome? Hematology. American Society of Hematology. Education Program, 2019(1): 426–432. doi: 10.1182/ HEMATOLOGY.2019000073.

Shah, A. et al. (2022). Migratory birds as the vehicle of transmission of multi drug resistant extended spectrum β lactamase producing Escherichia fergusonii, an emerging zoonotic pathogen. Saudi Journal of Biological Sciences, 29(5): 3167–3176. doi: 10.1016/J.SJBS.2022.01.057.

Sharma, A. et al. (2021). COVID-19: A Review on the Novel Coronavirus Disease Evolution, Transmission, Detection, Control and Prevention. Viruses, 13(2): 202. doi: 10.3390/V13020202.

Sharma, M. and Chakrabarti, A. (2020). On the origin of *Candida auris*: Ancestor, environmental stresses, and antiseptics. mBio, 11(6): 1–7. doi: 10.1128/MBIO.02102-20.

Sidhwa, F. and Itani, K.M.F. (2015). Skin preparation before surgery: Options and evidence. Surgical Infections, 16(1): 14–23. doi: 10.1089/SUR.2015.010.

Smith, D.J. et al. (2013). Intercontinental dispersal of bacteria and archaea by transpacific winds. Applied and Environmental Microbiology. 79(4): 1134-9. doi: 10.1128/AEM.03029-12.

Strand, T.M. and Lundkvist, Å. (2019). Rat-borne diseases at the horizon. A systematic review on infectious agents carried by rats in Europe 1995–2016. Infection Ecology & Epidemiology, 9(1). doi: 10.1080/20008686.2018.1553461.

Su, Q. and Liu, Q. (2021). Factors affecting gut microbiome in daily diet. Frontiers in Nutrition, 8: 218. doi: 10.3389/FNUT.2021.644138/BIBTEX.

Svärd, S.G. et al. (2003). Giardia lamblia—a model organism for eukaryotic cell differentiation. FEMS Microbiology Letters, 218(1): 3–7. doi: 10.1111/J.1574-6968.2003.TB11490.X.

Taylor, M. and Raja, A. (2022). Oral Candidiasis. Treasure Island: StatPearls Publishing.

Tello, J. et al. (2019). Major Outbreaks in the Nineteenth Century Shaped Grape Phylloxera Contemporary Genetic Structure in Europe. Scientific Reports, 9(1): 1–11. doi: 10.1038/s41598-019-54122-0.

Temmam, S. et al. (2022). Bat coronaviruses related to SARS-CoV-2 and infectious for human cells. Nature, 604(7905): 330–336. doi: 10.1038/s41586-022-04532-4.

Thèves, C. et al. (2016). History of smallpox and its spread in human populations. in paleomicrobiology of humans. Microbiol Spectr, 4(4): 161–172. doi: 10.1128/microbiolspec.poh-0004-2014.

Trigos, A.S. et al. (2018). How the evolution of multicellularity set the stage for cancer. British Journal of Cancer, 118(2): 145–152. doi: 10.1038/bjc.2017.398.

Tuite, A.R. et al. (2018). Infectious disease implications of large-scale migration of Venezuelan nationals. Journal of Travel Medicine, 25(1). doi: 10.1093/JTM/TAY077.

USDA APHIS Spotted Lanternfly (no date). Available at: https://www.aphis.usda.gov/aphis/resources/ pests-diseases/hungry-pests/slf/spotted-lanternfly (Accessed: 20 April 2022).

Vepštaitė-Monstavičė, I. et al. (2018). Saccharomyces paradoxus K66 Killer System Evidences Expanded Assortment of Helper and Satellite Viruses. Viruses, 10(10): 564. doi: 10.3390/V10100564.

Vogwill, T. and MacLean, R.C. (2015). The genetic basis of the fitness costs of antimicrobial resistance: a meta-analysis approach. Evolutionary Applications, 8(3): 284. doi: 10.1111/EVA.12202.

Volland, J.-M. et al. (2022). A centimeter-long bacterium with DNA compartmentalized in membrane-bound organelles. Science. 2022 Jun 24; 376(6600): 1453–1458. doi: 10.1126/science.abb3634.

Walker, J.W. et al. (2018). Transmissibility of emerging viral zoonoses. PLoS ONE, 13(11). doi: 10.1371/ journal.pone.0206926.

Walters, M.J. (2014). Birds, Pigs, and People: The Rise of Pandemic Flus. Seven Modern Plagues, 2014: 151–173. doi: 10.5822/978-1-61091-466-6_7.

Wehrs, M. et al. (2019). Engineering robust production microbes for large-scale cultivation. Trends in Microbiology, 27(6): 524–537. doi: 10.1016/J.TIM.2019.01.006.

Willems, H.M.E. et al. (2020). Vulvovaginal Candidiasis: A Current Understanding and Burning Questions. Journal of fungi Basel, 6(1). doi: 10.3390/JOF6010027.

Wilson, P. (2016). Microbiological surveillance in the critically ill. *In:* Webb, A. et al. (eds.). Oxford Textbook of Critical Care. Oxford University Press. doi: 10.1093/med/9780199600830.003.0281.

Wooley, J.C. et al. (2010). A Primer on Metagenomics. PLoS Computational Biology. Public Library of Science, 6(2): e1000667. doi: 10.1371/JOURNAL.PCBI.1000667.

Xing, Z. et al. (2020). Innate immune memory of tissue-resident macrophages and trained innate immunity: Re-vamping vaccine concept and strategies. Journal of Leukocyte Biology, 108(3): 825–834. doi: 10.1002/JLB.4MR0220-446R.

Yang, G. et al. (2020). Ssu72 regulates fungal development, aflatoxin biosynthesis and pathogenicity in *Aspergillus flavus*. Toxins, 12(11): 717. doi: 10.3390/TOXINS12110717.

Yang, X.L. et al. (2021). The intestinal microbiome primes host innate immunity against enteric virus systemic infection through type I interferon. mBio, 12(3). doi: 10.1128/MBIO.00366-21/SUPPL_FILE/MBIO.00366-21-ST001.DOCX.

Zalla, L.C. et al. (2022). Racial/Ethnic and age differences in the direct and indirect effects of the COVID-19 pandemic on US mortality. American Journal of Public Health, 112(1): 154–164. doi: 10.2105/AJPH.2021.306541.

6

The Enemy Within
Turning the Pages

M.E. Kambouris[1] *and Y. Manoussopoulos*[2,*]

Introduction

Individual cells creating populations or communities is the socio-ecological basis of unicellularity, with further integration achieved as one moves upwards, to different levels of the microbiome (Kambouris and Velegraki 2020). On the other hand, multicellularity seems rather well-defined: it is regularly attributed to cases where cells are in physical and functional continuity (Gilbert et al. 2012, Arendt et al. 2016, Tetz and Tetz 2020). The 'physical' by itself is not enough, as different individuals/cells may find themselves in close proximity due to environmental factors, as in herding, swarming, stampeding or surging, a condition which may cause some degree of interaction—from exchange of genetic material to differences in behavior or physiology, such as perspiration, rise of temperature and sexual reflexes.

Thus, to define an aggregation of cells as a multicellular organism, functional attributes would be pursued, and this must be done with extreme caution. The issue of cellular communication is indicative: in its simplest form, cellular communication is implemented by the exchange of chemical signals and products/by-products through different categories of membrane transportation infrastructure (Ahmed and Xiang 2011). Still, in highly evolved multicellular organisms, cells communicate and interact directly and in a precisely coordinated manner, without physical contact. The paradigm of such 'long-range transcellular communication' is the secretions from endocrine glands; the whole concept being a subcase of 'non-contact cell-to-cell interactions', which include the toxic effects of secreted toxins.

[1] University of Patras, School of Health Sciences, Department of Pharmacy, Patras, Greece & The Golden Helix Foundation, London, United Kingdom.
Email: mekambouris@yahoo.com, ORCID iD: https://orcid.org/0000-0002-3205-4797
[2] ELGO-Demeter, Plant Protection Division of Patras, Patras, Greece.
* Crresponding author: inminz@gmail.com, ORCID iD: https://orcid.org/0000-0002-6065-7368

Communication of information (or rather data) by such secretions *is* a transcellular signaling pathway. There are still some issues with the definition, given that the cells of a multicellular organism are highly and diversely differentiated and still interact by transcellular, long-range pathways through (bio)chemical means.

Primarily, a working, integrative criterion must be defined to pinpoint the mechanistic difference between the abovementioned concept of multicellular setup and the members of a colony that operate in similar if not identical terms and conditions. In both cases, there is a homeostasis function, which tends to conserve a *status quo* or to abide by a developmental blueprint. The latter, in turn, requires a spatiotemporal orientation system, a requirement resolved by quorum-sensing mechanisms. Another prerogative is the development of a recognition system that identifies similar or at least compatible units (cells) and distinguishes them from aliens—a prerequisite for individuality (Kourilsky 2016).

Subsequently, the multicellular concept can include some form of enforced choices for the "Greater Good" in the form of making and implementing executive decisions that benefit the whole of the community at the expense of some individuals. The Programmed Cell Death (PCD), known as apoptosis in multicellular organisms, is one such process. There is bacterial PCD, indicatively but not exclusively in the processes of sporulation and biofilm formation (Hammer 2018). The Enforced Suicide to cause minimal disruption and further follow-on processes in a tidy and neat manner is an indication of high-order integration and could prove useful in a variety of conditions, for it not only increases the resilience of the collective, but also allows differentiated processes with optimal energy expenditure and relatively limited allocation of regulation resources.

Furthermore, the line between a society and a complex living organism is anything but well-defined—the bioentities or members of the former may be considered simply higher-order cells of a given species (*sensu lato*) of the latter. Genomic identity is also precarious. So, where does the status of 'variance' change to 'difference'? The definition of a turning point in terms of integrative biology, where a community integrates or transitions into an organism, similar to the sociological threshold whence a group becomes a community, is of quintessential importance. More to the point, a core event must be identified. One that changes the attitude, social and biochemical, from an individualized to collective mode of life, susceptible to some form of administration, possibly but not necessarily featuring morphological and functional transformation.

Moreover, as a consequence of the above, the idea of a nameless multitude of surging cells is perhaps oversimplistic. Hence, a notion of germ-ganism (Kambouris et al. 2022) should be considered, according to which these cell populations are parts of, or strive to establish, a multicellular entity—a germ-ganism—with regulatory and diverse development/ontogeny and self-restrain growth functions. This is applicable to both transient populations and founder cells that may emerge from a contamination event, or are members of the existing microbiomes. To make things more complicated, multi-microbial microbiomes, like the ones colonizing different biocompartments of macroorganisms, may be found in different cases of diseases instead of homogenous populations of individual species. It is thus natural to assume that the causal pathogen in case of a disease may be assisted by other members of the microbiome, not pathogenic by themselves but pivotal for either the pathogenic attitude of the pathogen proper (compared to a possible benign colonization) or the success of the infectious process and resilience of the pathogen, or both.

Last, but not least, the pathogen *is* a foreign entity (no biochemical signaling identity, no administrative integration), but this should be taken *sensu lato*: tumors are not germs, but they are apperceived by the host as alien entities. They actually act as such, meaning they define themselves, plausibly tacitly, as a different, distinct entity with interests conflicting with the ones of the host, contrary to the attitude adopted by well-adapted parasites towards their host.

Eukaryotic and prokaryotic germ-ganisms

Form and function do not necessarily go hand-in-hand. There are cases where implementing a different routine due to an environmental trigger does not result in any appreciable morphological change that could count as transformation. Such cases include hibernation in large animals (Geiser 2013) and the swarm mode in grasshoppers (Sword et al. 2000, Rogers et al. 2003). It is possible that the highly evolved and complex body forms of higher organisms are adequate, if not suitable, in order to satisfy the functional specifications of alternative routines. This does not take into account the sheer complexity and difficulty in energy demands and programming for altering sophisticated bodyforms regularly and rapidly in order to respond to such triggers in the abovementioned cases. One-off changes, on the other hand, as in the successive transformation stages of the ontogeny of insects, are perfectly doable and the field of embryology contains a huge collection of such transformations and events of gradual and successive but irreversible (as a rule) adaptation to demanding situations and complex functional blueprints. It must be noted that the reversal to stem cells, spontaneous (as in lower animals) or stimulated (as with the once popular biotechnological therapeutic approach), belies the clause of irreversibility.

Fungi supreme: The exemplary germ-ganisms

Binary fission of cells is applicable to both mycelial and colonial forms of fungi. Even then, yeast cells (implying the unicellular, planktonic form of some higher-taxa fungi that, when propagating at a steady position, forms colonies) follow a different propagation mechanism—the budding, a version of the fission but resulting in unequal parts. It actually produces daughter cells (one at each procreation event) from maternal cells but the latter remain as such: the process is not one mother cell producing two identical daughter cells, but one mother cell producing one, smaller and fast-growing daughter cell at a time. The mother cell remains adult, without revamping its physiology and bear scars identifying the location of the procreation event; according to a number of factors a mother cell may produce further offspring or not (Beran 1968).

Budding of yeasts is in effect a branching process with less suppression enacted. A rather accurate description of budding using branching terminology might be 'multiple *branching* events of one step each, following a much more liberal 3-D pattern in spatial terms but never coexisting in the same temporal frame'. Some yeasts form pseudohyphae and certain higher fungi are occasionally endowed with the ability to change their physiology and alter their appearance, transforming into different thallic forms. This phenomenon, when unfolding between the two basic forms, the mycelial multicellular one (suitable for local growth) and the colonial unicellular one (suitable for dispersion, mainly in liquid environments), is called dimorphism. Dimorphic fungi have both yeast and true hyphal phases (Gow and Gooday 1982a,b). Moreover, the peculiar propagation of *Schizosaccharomyces*, by fission rather than budding (Mitchison 1990), is halfway the evolutionary distance between yeast cells and mycelium thallic systems, for it combines the daughter cell separation of the former with the spatial self-restriction of the latter. With all this in mind, observations of both thallic systems should be viewed preferentially through expansive criteria; however, projections to other living forms of bacteria, animalia and plantae should not be disregarded.

The mycelial configuration of a fungal cell is different from that of the unicellular one of the same, dimorphic fungal species (Calderone and Fonzi 2001) and the transformation may occur through a chemical or thermal, or any other, environmental trigger. When growing in mycelia, fungi (may) develop differentiated structures, occasionally deploying organs, especially reproductive organs or fruiting bodies (e.g., mushrooms), and show elaborate morphologies even in petri dish (Figure 6.1A-D). When in a colonial state with unicellular formats, such characteristics are much less prominent, but they *do* appear. A relevant example here is that of yeasts which grow colonies, not mycelia; but the form of the said colonies (*switch phenotypes*, namely smooth, irregular, fuzzy or stipple) is peculiar (Velegraki et al. 1996) and may change over time with environmental conditions (Velegraki 1995) and time (and thus, age). This diversity in colonial, and not merely cellular, phenotype simply implies a pattern of arranging cells in space and time, even without functional integration. As a result, different genomic routines are triggered to allow the formation of different phenotypes, a hypothesis proven in the case of switching cell phenotypes from white to opaque (Brimacombe et al. 2020). This introduces the notion of 'pseudo-mycelia' (Palková and Váchová 2016). It refers to a conglomeration of hyphae wherein the cells forming these hyphae are not functionally integrated. They are arranged in linear succession and touch, or rather stick to each other, but are not differentiated as in true hyphae and do not exhibit intercellular communication by biomass streaming through pores. They remain separated by double cell envelope, one part from each adjoining cell, contrary to the septa arrangement of true hyphae. The exchange is through proper membranic channels and cell wall chokepoints, thus creating a morphology similar to hyphae, but of less or no functional integration (Váchová et al. 2012), a good rationale for the name 'pseudohyphae' (Vallejo et al. 2013). It is important to note that neither pseudomycelia nor mycelia by definition show the embedment of cells in an extracellular matrix. Cells may be differentiated in structure and shape according to the multi- or unicellular routine implemented at any given time, but extracellular matrices are not a given. As is the case with switching phenotypes, pseudomycelia are an intermediate state of cellular organization, exhibiting more dedicated spatial positioning than the one seen in plain colonial

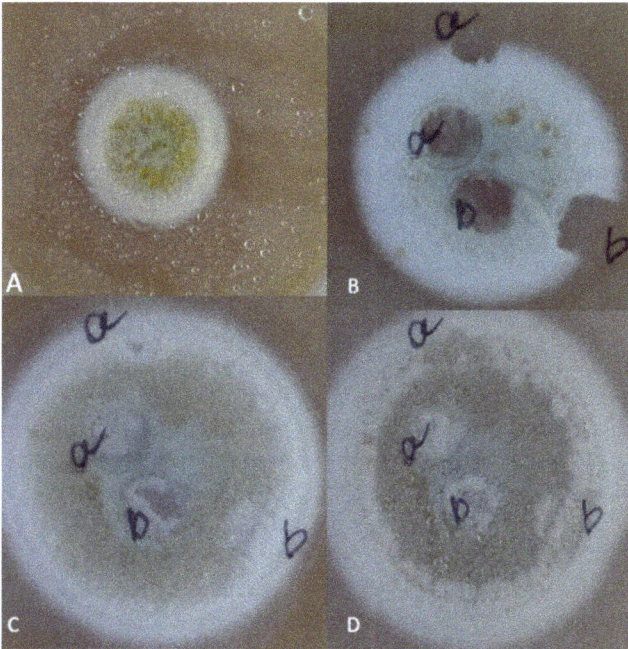

Figure 6.1. (B) The sites of surface punches collected from the periphery and from intermediate positions of a *Penicillium* sp. mycelial mat show (C) evident healing in 1 day. (A) The undisturbed, concurrent control may be used for comparison, to make evident the concentric texture and color differentiation due to age. (D) In 2 days, healing is complete, but the difference between the new and the original mycelium is obvious with patches in the case of the former. Patches in the periphery are more integrated into the surrounding mycelium in terms of morphology than patches near the center of the mycelium. Which remain visually distinct.

formats, but with no differentiation, physiological integration and intertwining as is observed in true multicellular formats like mycelia (Palková and Váchová 2016).

The key here is to understand that proximity is important. Mycelia may occur in liquid cultures, manifesting their characteristics, but pseudomycelia and switch phenotypes of colonies generally do not; in liquids, the unattached cells do not keep their assigned positions and are not under constant surveillance by a fixed population of neighbors and peers (Kourilsky 2016). Thus, subject to viscosity and fluid dynamics, planktonic cells remain independent and their dynamics simple.

But not *that* simple. If unicellular organisms are inoculated in a plate and incubated under suboptimal conditions, their growth is slower than in optimal conditions. What is more important, the said growth stops spontaneously, despite ample nutrients and room for further expansion in the petri dish; the inclusion of humidity factors in the inoculation chamber ensures that the substrate does not dry out and, thus, local draught is not a factor. Consequently, in a colonial format, the organism does not grow indefinitely even if external conditions nominally allow it. Growth reaches some spatial limitation, which may differ with varying degrees of environmental suitability, ranging from total growth suspension to optimization. It is unknown whether such limits do or do not exist in optimal conditions, or simply fall far outside the scope and margins of current experimental procedures and instrumentation. For example, if the limitation occurs when the radial expansion is over 20 cm, there are no petri dishes available to conduct experiments. Consequently, the growth would terminate forcibly at the edges of the dish and would give the impression of spontaneously unlimited growing dynamics. Similarly, if one takes into consideration that fungi, in mycelial format, may spread over several meters in nature and produce clusters of mushrooms growing from the same subterranean mycelial network, the issue of distance becomes clear. However, it cannot be determined whether the expansion of such a mycelium stopped because it reached the spatial edge of permissive environment, or due to a preordained range of development and growth.

The nature of the arrest signal(s) is quintessential, and possibly of quorum-sensing nature (Dunny et al. 2008, Costa-Orlandi et al. 2017, Whalen et al. 2019). Such signaling can be produced by metabolites released continuously, not cleared and locally accumulating, when their concentration or sheer volume reaches a threshold. It could be a one-off or reversible switch, its exact nature depending on the phase of the growth curve. For example, cultures of streaked isolates of *S. aureus* growing at 35°C on nutrient agar stopped growing spontaneously after 72 hours. But a sample taken from this arrested culture and streaked on to another petri dish with fresh substrate grew normally for 48 hours, and the growth remained unchanged at 72 hours; however, in the sampled area, no growth occurred to recover the emptied space (Figure 6.2). Obviously, the arrest signal, quorum-sensing or otherwise, persists on the spot and inhibits resumption of growth. This may be combined with the possibility that the cells of the culture as a whole already moved to a stable state, a growth plateau, and could not revert to the active status, although in this case the extracted sample would not have grown when moved to a fresh dish either.

On the contrary, centrally inoculated cultures of mycelial fungi, when punch-sampled in a similar manner (Figure 6.1A), show secondary growth that covers the depleted areas as a patch-on (Figure 6.1D). Healing tissue is ultimately (in the 5th day) fully incorporated and visually undistinguishable from the surrounding, original tissue in the case of edge punches, but observably different from the surrounding tissue in the inner extraction locations. Although the patches were fully integrated physically, as they grew from the periphery towards the center, they did not catch up to

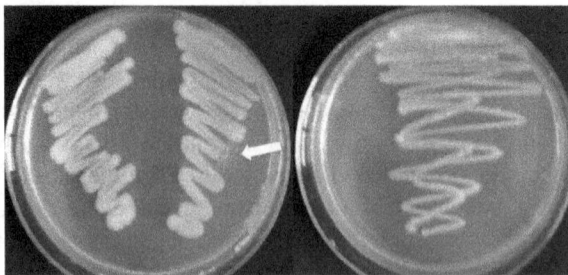

Figure 6.2. *Staphylococcus aureus* streaked and grown on nutrient agar at 35°C. (Left) Initial culture, in duplicate; sampled area shown clearly by arrow. The subtracted biomass has not been replaced after 3 days, thus indicating showing developmental stasis, whereas (Right) the subtracted biomass, in the same time shows standard growth when transferred in new and chemically/environmetally identical environment.

the developmental phase by the 8th day (when the experiment was discontinued due to secondary growth). The patches differed in morphology (color-texture) from the surrounding mycelium, the difference being more prominent towards the center and the older, more ancient biomass/hyphae and less prominent towards the periphery. When the experiment was repeated with the source mycelium having grown to the physical limit of the dish and thus at growth arrest, the excised tissue did grow on new dishes but was not replaced by patches of new growth at the points of excision, even after five weeks had elapsed. Thus, it can be concluded that the mycelium heals the loss of tissue/biomass when punch-sampled during its active growth; it does not heal when punch-sampled after entering the growth plateau or stasis, although the excised samples do retain their vitality and grow if transplanted into new dishes, indicating a reversible growth arrest.

The tissues, organs and limps of higher-order animals or plants do not grow uncontrollably, but reach certain spatial limitations (which differ within the species and due to different numbers of produced cells and not to difference in size of the cells forming the organ). Thus, accepting such a programming precaution for a fungus is not a cognitive overextension in any way; multicellular structures seem to develop in fungi when the growth is arrested and cells are in a static phase, where differentiation may occur due to differential expression (Palková and Váchová 2016). It is admittedly a much cruder example of planning, compared to the elaborate blueprints the ontogenies of mammals implement, but a set plan nevertheless, followed by the organism.

Biofilms: A compound form of germ-ganism

In many tissues, the cells of multicellular organisms are embedded in an extracellular matrix, produced by the cells themselves and usually complemented by inorganic residues absorbed from the environment and placed within the structure following some logic or pattern, with or without prior processing. Alternatively, inorganic residues may be incorporated directly into the matrix as the latter is secreted or excreted by the cell into the environment, without prior absorption by the cell, despite the biological and structural complications in the acquisition and arrangement of the said elements. If the cells in such a format (the bone being an excellent example) are considered as a part of one organ and organism, there is no reason to believe that this is not applicable to microbiota within a single species and genomically homogenous biofilm (Neu and Lawrence 2014, Patrinos et al. 2020). Within the bone structure, cells are at a steady though occasionally varying distance from each other and communicate only through the matrix material. This probably occurs by chemical signals, but other formats may be applicable with different kinds of waves, transmittable through dense mass (Kourilsky 2016). Similarly, cells attached on the basement membrane, a standard in many tissues (especially but not exclusively epithelia) of multicellular organisms are arranged in a 2-D setting and constitute a subcase of cells embedded within a matrix. The basement membrane is a residual but highly organized matrix which is relatively thin and deployed to just one side of the cells, as the latter are densely packed adjacent to each other and connected by tight junctions, desmosomes and gap junctions, which create intracellular polarity that results in functional optimization across the gradient of the said polarity.

A biofilm is essentially "…a hydrated 3-D structure of cells and extracellular polymeric substance" (Neu and Lawrence 2014) and very similar to the concept of basement membrane plus attached cells. The sessile forms of microbiota which are embedded in a biofilm differ from the respective planktonic forms, which is the definition of dimorphism by biotic style (Nadal et al. 2008, Rollet et al. 2009, van Wolferen et al. 2018), an equivalent of the multimorphic differentiation of cells by tissue and type in multicellular organisms. All the cells of a multicellular organism (notwithstanding chimerae and mosaicism) share the same functional blueprints and directives hardwired into their genomes. However, the implementation of different routines is obvious and of both spatial and temporal nature, meaning that it depends on the cell type and the development phase of the cells and the organism. The former differentiation means that the multimorphism is concurrent, with different forms occurring simultaneously. On the contrary, sequential dimorphism occurs in specific cases in multicellular organisms, as in ontogenesis; however, in unicellular organisms, it is the only mode of multimorphism, dictated by conditions and triggered by some signal. At the reception of the latter, all cells transform and change their functional profile downstream from the transcriptome to the metabolome and secretome, especially in quantitative terms. However, they retain normativity in the collective level and recognize and communicate with each other (Kourilsky 2016) and also exhibit a collective sort of homeostasis to an extent.

There are highly heterogenous biofilms, multi-microbial in nature, where cells of different species coexist (Patrinos et al. 2020), cells of different kingdoms or even domains of life occasionally. This may be taken as an evolutionary advantageous characteristic, since "diversity is an asset prospectively safeguarding from Chance events" (Kourilsky 2016). This inclusive character of biofilms is reminiscent of the definition of a chimera (Malan et al. 2006, De Los Angeles 2020) if the biofilm is taken as an organism with cells exclusively carrying multiple genomes and communicating from afar by exchanging signals through the matrix. This suggests a chimeric germ-ganism.

Admittedly, chimeras are usually a matter of different pedigrees rather than species; the different genomes of a chimera are variants of the same species. Still, the aforementioned notion of multimicrobial biofilms being considered chimeric germ-ganisms does not stretch the issue too thin: a loose definition based on the original Greek *Chimera* monster (a tripartite hybrid of goat, lion and bird—all higher animals, it must be stressed) allows and actually encourages more inclusive and broad interpretations; thus chimeras of cells of different species are a legitimate concept.

In any case, the inclusion of cells of different *kingdoms* or even *domains* in one organism may be pushing these conventions to the limit. Once intercellular physical distance and physical contact are no more the defining qualities of an organism as opposed to a community, the genomic homogeneity can be understood to be the next definitional step. Unfortunately, the idea of an organism being genetically homogenous and that of society being inclusive of diversity is a bit misleading and not clear-cut.

For starters, societies are not necessarily inclusive. Societies that are by definition open to different species, races and even pedigrees/tribes are a rather modern contraption, and societies *may* be very exclusive and homogenous and have been so in numerous historic and biological examples across spatial and temporal expanses. This is suggested by sociological, historical/anthropological and even ethological/zoological data, bees being a perfect example. The pedigree, which equals to genomic homogeneity, is considered a defining character not just of individuals, but of communities as well. The fact that high degrees of consanguinity were not unknown, nor discouraged in many historical periods and cultures, substantiates striving for exclusivity and homogeneity. On the other hand, transgenic organisms (genomes of different species artificially merged into the same nucleus) blur the lines of genomic homogeneity in an individual, although this issue is materially and conceptually irrelevant to biofilms.

As a result, the demarcation between aggregation/society and organism has been fuzzy for some three decades. This was long before the concept of microbiome produced a paradigm shift, by introducing the notion of the holobiont, described as the "sum of the macro-organism and its appendage (sub)microbiomes situated in different biocompartments" (Patrinos et al. 2020). Consequently, the wildly different genomes present in a multispecies or even multidomain biofilm do not forbid its inclusion in the germ-ganism concept if the latter is applied expansively.

The tumor-ganism

Infections caused by the deregulation of the appendage microbiomes of a multicellular macroorganism/host, and other such conditions, are conceptually similar to cancer, where strictly native cells are deregulated, alienated in terms of genome, regulation and communication protocols (Kourilsky 2016) and ultimately become detrimental or a threat to the balance achieved by some (central, decentralized or even dispersed) control authority. The tumor is genomically heterogeneous as it may be made up of many primary lesions coming into contact and combining. Each lesion may be produced by a different (in terms of target location, temporal distribution or causative agent) carcinogenic event. Additionally, even the clonal cells produced by uncontrollable propagation in a lesion vary wildly in genomic terms due to the patent genetic instability, an added consequence of the causative deregulation (Burrell et al. 2013). Taking the above into account, each tumor may be also considered as a tumor-ganism. An integrated approach to the possible interplay and interrelation between different (surging or metastasizing) tumors in one macroorganism/host would be of immense interest. Tumors are brought to stasis and have cells or groups of cells (persisters) that are more important than others and, thus, better protected or more resilient, occasionally in functional hypnosis to avoid detrimental exchanges with the environment (Swayden et al. 2020). If the standard cells are depleted, the persisters become activated and produce new cells to replenish the ranks, thus causing a relapse. This has direct microbiomics equivalents (Iskandar et al. 2022), implying a universal mode of organization for seemingly non-affiliated cell aggregations.

A viral equivalent: The "Sur-ganism"

Viruses have only recently, and still far from unanimously, been considered as living organisms (Pearson 2008, Desnues et al. 2012). Thus, functions such as intentional combination, task management and procedural exemplification are not the favorite areas of study for researchers. Viruses cannot be seen to form higher-order organisms, by any definition, no matter how loose, as they cannot integrate in higher forms that would require or/and exhibit homeostasis, which is one of the prerequisites for individuality (Kourilsky 2016). Still, there is an intrinsic possibility that they follow swarming rather than surging attack protocols when in a host-rich environment. It is well understood that a single cell is expected to be assaulted by a number of virions overwhelming cellular defences. The exact values differ by cell type and status and vary among different virus types and, possibly, strains. Of course, there are *optima*—when assaulted by too many virions, a cell may collapse before releasing new viruses; this explains why virally infected cells may be rendered inaccessible or invulnerable to other and subsequent virus assaults through Viral Interference (Dianzani 1975, Yang et al. 2021). This increases the host population that may be infected by a given number of virions and has the added advantage of not allowing additional virion ingress after a threshold is reached. In effect, (re)shuffling of parts and genomes of different viruses within the same cell becomes less probable. Such reshuffling may fuel evolution but surely results in many defective virions being produced due to recombination events of various parts—not only genomes, but also proteins may interfere with each other during the assembly of new virions, thus greatly diminishing the output of spawn.

In such a context, it is possible that the virions, when approaching a target population, do not follow stochastic patterns for approaching and attempting docking with specific cells. It may be a chaotic event, as thought of generally, with the peculiars still unresolved, which could be studied by non-destructive dyes and atomic force or scanning probe microscopy. But what is often bypassed is the possibility that, in this event, there is a pattern similar to the swarming practices of higher organisms. This aspect has been overlooked as it is considered an impossibility once the virus is known to have neither self-cognition nor communication abilities—both are essential for decision-making and assignment allocation processes inherent to swarming, which would be expected to optimize the assault ratio in order to maximize infection success and efficiency of dispersion in the host population (Choudoir et al. 2018). The latter is required to be as fast and voluminous as possible, to evade or rather outpace collective cellular countermeasures as the ones induced by interferon secretion.

A passive swarming logic would be that changes within a cell infected and overrun by virions include alterations in surface characteristics and thus discourage virions arriving late from docking on to the nearest cells, which would be already infected, and make them advance in terms of space farther within the host population to find benign, preferably totally unaffected, cells. This is the simplest pattern; others are conceivable as well, but would require higher order of perception, occasionally self-awareness and definitely decision-making. The passive swarming could be affected under some form of automation ingrained into the virions—from a balance of attraction and repulsion among them to create a cut-off threshold in density, to funneling following virions past if not away from the successfully infected cells, but possibly not from assaulted but not successfully infected ones, such as the ones docked by virions in numbers below the infectious threshold.

Conclusion

The microbial flora has long been identified as a key factor in the development of infections, both by (a) supplying pathogens, in active (obligatory pathogens) or inactive form (induced stasis or hypobiosis, including but not limited to cysts, spores and sclerotia, or naturally selected low virulence strains or opportunistic/facultative pathogens), and (b) suppressing/regulating them (Valentin-Weigand 2005, Paul et al. 2019, Vlaar et al. 2021). The latter is a very heterogeneous phenomenon, the effect of a number of causes occurring individually or in any combination, with the collective effect being unpredictable. The antagonism of microbial species is one such cause, possibly the most important.

By progressing to the notion of the microbiome (Kambouris and Velegraki 2020), interactions are understood as more integrated. The notion suggests a collective entity, not an aggregation of (dis)similar individuals as in 'flora'. The standard of the said interactions refers to benign constant exchange with the host, the latter being, more or less, the environment of the microbiota of the microbiome and not a friendly giant occasionally used by some rapacious microbiota within the tribe as pray and ground for exploitation. The germ-ganism (Kambouris et al. 2022) suggests higher-order integration within the microbiome, endowed with additional functions occurring not as a reaction to a causative event, but cognitively, to achieve some ends. Whether this is the result of some dispersed, distributed intelligence not yet decoded or the result of interwoven decision loops with feedback in a purely mechanistic form is yet to be determined. But the germ-ganism does introduce a reactionary concept, possibly responsible for the failure of the efforts to manipulate pathogens. This must have been effected by cognitive, if not intelligent, sensing, deciding and responding. Additionally, the use of helper microbiota to support or even enhance the direct action of the openly pathogenic ones needs to be seriously considered.

A very distant concept is that of persister cells, which do not help the colony/population/microbiome to thrive, evolve or expand, but ensure the collective survival—as opposed to eradication—when under extreme conditions, including but not restricted to exposure to antimicrobials of various kinds, especially (bio) chemicals (Sulaiman and Lam 2021, Iskandar et al. 2022). In any case, the concept of the pathobiome (Berg et al. 2020), a subcase of a holobiome going astray, may well be preferentially interpreted under the light of the germ-ganism rather than of some spontaneous and unintended transformation from a mutualistic or commensalistic phase of the holobiont.

Thus, given that the microbiome holds the key to the development of pathogenicity, be that incoming or evolving (Kambouris et al. 2018, Kambouris et al. 2021), the germ-ganism may explain differences in the outcome of infection as well as of therapy, and account for the marked evolution of the infectivity, at large, against numerous, if not all, populations/species of interest within the humanome, but quite possibly beyond it and, why not, long before it. If the germ-ganism is a reality, it surely did not expect humans to emerge and the humanome to meddle with it.

References

Ahmed, K.A. and Xiang, J. (2011). Mechanisms of cellular communication through intercellular protein transfer. Journal of Cellular and Molecular Medicine, 15(7): 1458–1473. doi: 10.1111/J.1582-4934.2010.01008.X.

Arendt, D. et al. (2016). The origin and evolution of cell types. Nature Reviews Genetics, 17(12): 744–757. doi: 10.1038/nrg.2016.127.

Beran, K. (1968). Budding of yeast cells, their scars and ageing. Advances in Microbial Physiology, 2: 143–171.

Berg, G. et al. (2020). Microbiome definition re-visited: Old concepts and new challenges. Microbiome, 8(1): 103. doi: 10.1186/s40168-020-00875-0.

Brimacombe, C.A. et al. (2020). A white-to-opaque-like phenotypic switch in the yeast Torulaspora microellipsoides. Communications Biology, 3(1). doi: 10.1038/S42003-020-0815-6.

Burrell, R.A. et al. (2013). The causes and consequences of genetic heterogeneity in cancer evolution. Nature, 501(7467): 338–345. doi: 10.1038/nature12625.

Calderone, R.A. and Fonzi, W.A. (2001). Virulence factors of *Candida albicans*. Trends in Microbiology, 9(7): 327–335. doi: 10.1016/S0966-842X(01)02094-7.

Choudoir, M.J. et al. (2018). Variation in range size and dispersal capabilities of microbial taxa. Ecology. Ecology, 99(2): 322–334. doi: 10.1002/ECY.2094.

Costa-Orlandi, C.B. et al. (2017). Fungal biofilms and polymicrobial diseases. Journal of Fungi (Basel, Switzerland), 3(2): 22. doi: 10.3390/jof3020022.

Desnues, C. et al. (2012). Sputnik, a virophage infecting the viral domain of life. pp. 63–89. *In*: Advances in Virus Research. Academic Press Inc. doi: 10.1016/B978-0-12-394621-8.00013-3.

Dianzani, F. (1975). Viral interference and interferon. La Ricerca in clinica e in laboratorio, 5(3): 196–213. doi: 10.1007/BF02908284.

Dunny, G. et al. (2008). Multicellular behavior in bacteria: Communication, cooperation, competition and cheating. BioEssays : News and Reviews in Molecular, Cellular and Developmental Biology, 30(4): 296–298. doi: 10.1002/BIES.20740.

Geiser, F. (2013). Hibernation. Current Biology, 23(5). doi: 10.1016/j.cub.2013.01.062.

Gilbert, S.F. et al. (2012). A symbiotic view of life: We have never been individuals.Quarterly Review of Biology, 87(4): 325–341. doi: 10.1086/668166.

Gow, N.A.R. and Gooday, G.W. (1982a). Growth kinetics and morphology of colonies of the filamentous form of Candida albicans. Journal of General Microbiology, 128(9): 2187–2194. doi: 10.1099/00221287-128-9-2187.

Gow, N.A.R. and Gooday, G.W. (1982b). Vacuolation, branch production and linear growth of germ tubes of *Candida albicans*. Journal of General Microbiology, 128(9): 2195–2198. doi: 10.1099/00221287-128-9-2195.

Hammer, N.D. (2018). Microbial programmed cell death. Apoptosis and Beyond: The Many Ways Cells Die. John Wiley & Sons, Ltd, pp. 49–70. doi: 10.1002/9781119432463.CH3.

Iskandar, K. et al. (2022). Antibiotic Discovery and Resistance: The Chase and the Race. Antibiotics, 11(2): 182. doi: 10.3390/ANTIBIOTICS11020182.

Kambouris, M. and Velegraki, A. (2020). Introduction: The Microbiome as a concept: Vogue or necessity? pp. 1–4. *In*: Kambouris, M.E. and Velegraki, A. (eds.). Microbiomics: Dimensions, Applications, and Translational Implications of Human and Environmental Microbiome Research. 1st edn. Elsevier Academic Press.

Kambouris, M.E. et al. (2018). Humanome versus microbiome: games of dominance and pan-biosurveillance in the Omics Universe. OMICS A Journal of Integrative Biology, 22(8): 528–538. doi: 10.1089/omi.2018.0096.

Kambouris, M.E., Manoussopoulos, Y. and Velegraki, A. (2021). The emerging pathogens: Nature, status, and threat. In Genomics in Biosecurity. 1st edn. London: ELSEVIER ACADEMIC PRESS, pp. 61–74.

Kambouris, M.E. et al. (2022). Beyond the microbiome: Germ-ganism? An integrative idea for microbial existence, organization, growth, pathogenicity, and therapeutics. Omics : A Journal of Integrative Biology, 26(4): 204–217. doi: 10.1089/OMI.2022.0015.

Kourilsky, P. (2016). The natural defense system and the normative self model. F1000Research., 5: 797. doi: 10.12688/F1000RESEARCH.8518.1.

De Los Angeles, A. (2020). Parsing the pluripotency continuum in humans and non-human primates for interspecies chimera generation. Experimental Cell Research, 387(1). doi: 10.1016/J.YEXCR.2019.111747.

Malan, V. et al. (2006). Chimera and other fertilization errors. Clinical Genetics, 70(5): 363–373. doi: 10.1111/J.1399-0004.2006.00689.X.

Mitchison, J.M. (1990). The fission yeast, Schizosaccharomyces pombe. BioEssays : News and Reviews in Molecular, Cellular and Developmental Biology. Bioessays, 12(4): 189–191. doi: 10.1002/BIES.950120409.

Nadal, M. et al. (2008). Dimorphism in fungal plant pathogens. FEMS Microbiology Letters, 284(2): 127–134. doi: 10.1111/J.1574-6968.2008.01173.X.

Neu, T.R. and Lawrence, J.R. (2014). Investigation of microbial biofilm structure by laser scanning microscopy. Advances in Biochemical Engineering/Biotechnology, 146: 1–51. doi: 10.1007/10_2014_272.

Palková, Z. and Váchová, L. (2016). Yeast cell differentiation: Lessons from pathogenic and non-pathogenic yeasts. Seminars in Cell and Developmental Biology, 57: 110–119. doi: 10.1016/J.SEMCDB.2016.04.006.

Patrinos, G.P. et al. (2020). Bacteriome and Archaeome: The core family under the microbiomic roof. *In:* Kambouris, M. and Velegraki, A. (eds.). Microbiomics: Dimensions, Applications, and Translational Implications of Human and Environmental Microbiome Research. ELSEVIER ACADEMIC PRESS.

Paul, C. et al. (2019). Bacterial spores, from ecology to biotechnology. Advances in Applied Microbiology, 106: 79–111. doi: 10.1016/BS.AAMBS.2018.10.002.

Pearson, H. (2008). "Virophage" suggests viruses are alive. Nature, 454(7205): 677. doi: 10.1038/454677a.

Rogers, S. et al. (2003). Mechanosensory-induced behavioural gregarization in the desert locust Schistocerca gregaria. The Journal of Experimental Biology, 206(22): 3991–4002. doi: 10.1242/JEB.00648.

Rollet, C. et al. (2009). Biofilm-detached cells, a transition from a sessile to a planktonic phenotype: A comparative study of adhesion and physiological characteristics in *Pseudomonas aeruginosa.* FEMS Microbiology Letters, 290(2): 135–42. doi: 10.1111/j.1574-6968.2008.01415.x.

Sulaiman, J.E. and Lam, H. (2021). Evolution of bacterial tolerance under antibiotic treatment and its implications on the development of resistance. Frontiers in Microbiology, 12: 431. doi: 10.3389/FMICB.2021.617412/BIBTEX.

Swayden, M. et al. (2020). Tolerant/persister cancer cells and the path to resistance to targeted therapy. Cells, 9(12). doi: 10.3390/CELLS9122601.

Sword, G. et al. (2000). Density-dependent aposematism in the desert locust. Proceedings. Biological Sciences, 267(1438): 63–68. doi: 10.1098/RSPB.2000.0967.

Tetz, V.V and Tetz, G.V. (2020). A new biological definition of life. Biomolecular Concepts, 11(1): 1–6. doi: 10.1515/bmc-2020-0001.

Váchová, L. et al. (2012). Yeast colonies: A model for studies of aging, environmental adaptation, and longevity. Oxidative Medicine and Cellular Longevity, 2012: 601836. doi: 10.1155/2012/601836.

Valentin-Weigand, P. (2005). Intracellular invasion and persistence: Survival strategies of Streptococcus suis and *Mycobacterium avium* ssp. paratuberculosis. Berl Munch Tierarztl Wochenschr, 117(11-12): 459–63.

Vallejo, J. et al. (2013). Cell aggregations in yeasts and their applications. Applied Microbiology and Biotechnology, 97(6): 2305–2318. doi: 10.1007/S00253-013-4735-Y.

Velegraki, A. (1995). *In vitro* susceptibility to itraconazole and fluconazole of switch phenotypes of Candida albicans serotypes A and B, isolated from immunocompromised hosts. J Med Vet Mycol, 33(1): 83–85.

Velegraki, A. et al. (1996). Variable antifungal susceptibility of wild-type *Candida albicans* phenotypes from neutropenic hosts. European Journal of Clinical Microbiology & Infectious Diseases, 15(11): 854–860. doi: 10.1007/BF01691215.

Vlaar, L.E. et al. (2021). On the role of dauer in the adaptation of nematodes to a parasitic lifestyle. Parasites & Vectors, 14(1). doi: 10.1186/S13071-021-04953-6.

Whalen, K.E. et al. (2019). Bacterial alkylquinolone signaling contributes to structuring microbial communities in the ocean. Microbiome, 7(1): 93. doi: 10.1186/s40168-019-0711-9.

van Wolferen, M. et al. (2018). Archaeal biofilm formation. Nature Reviews Microbiology, 16(11): 699–713. doi: 10.1038/s41579-018-0058-4.

Yang, X.L. et al. (2021). The intestinal microbiome primes host innate immunity against enteric virus systemic infection through type I interferon. mBio, 12(3). doi: 10.1128/MBIO.00366-21/SUPPL_FILE/MBIO.00366-21-ST001.DOCX.

7

The Hope of Biologicals
Toxins, Microbiomes and Phages

M.E. Kambouris

Introduction

The germ theory of (infectious) disease was introduced by Kircher in 1658. The operative idea was that, when found in host tissues, small agents unseen by the naked eye, but detectable under the microscope, were the cause of diseases. These agents were found almost everywhere in the environment and were occasionally but not necessarily, nor universally, associated with disease. Projecting this line of thought further, infectious diseases are attributed to masses of pathogens (of cellular or acellular nature, but of biological rather than biochemical nature) *invading* the host and trying to establish themselves there, destroying it as a direct result. Consequently, toxicosis/poisoning is *not* an infection, but it may be part of one, playing a supportive role in most cases, that is, by assisting the pathogen to establish its presence.

The aforementioned destruction may be direct, due to septic and/or toxic mechanism (Kambouris et al. 2018) or indirect, as in immunologic overreaction/ hyperinflammatory response (Karavitis and Kovacs 2011), or a combination of both. The sequence of events is characterized by a mutually detrimental exchange of attrition effects, possibly complicated by long-range migration of the invading population through blood or any other circulating liquid (Benninger and Steiner 2018). In this concept, any form of intervention (bio)chemical, biological/ biopharmaceutical or radiological/radiopharmaceutical—or the use of any other conceivable kind of effector (Declerck 2012, Lang et al. 2020) is meant to increase the rate of incapacitating the microbial cells to levels manageable by the immune

University of Patras, School of Health Sciences, Department of Pharmacy, Patras, Greece & The Golden Helix Foundation, London, United Kingdom
Email: mekambouris@yahoo.com, ORCID iD: https://orcid.org/0000-0002-3205-4797

system of the host. The above makes the immunological dimension of an infection, and disease in general, quintessential in medical decision-making. Such intervention may be defined as 'indirectly therapeutic', for it helps in removing the cause, and 'terminally targetable', as it ideally destroys/incapacitates the end effectors of the infection process: the cells/virions and their possible toxic or supportive products, such as toxins. Additional targets may be microbial products supportive of microbial growth without being detrimental themselves; examples are hydrolytic enzymes produced to counter antimicrobial agents (Kaminskaia et al. 2000) and iron-collecting molecules (Schrettl and Haas 2011) being essential for the survival of the pathogen.

All therapeutic interventions may benefit from understanding the function of the pathogen in a more integrative manner where it may be understood as a migrating community simply striving to establish itself as a colony (the lesion) in a nutrient-rich environment (the host), the immunological reactions of which are *not* apperceived by the said immigrant as resistance, counteraction or any hostile attitude, but as a negative environmental incident—an equivalent of 'climate crisis' in terms and proportions of the microworld. Additionally, the pathogenic community might as well be there already and not *invading*, but *transforming* into a more aggressive, resource-hungry state and mode of development/expansion (Kambouris et al. 2021). Appendage microbiomes, not only of humans but also of animals and plants, are the perfect starter for an invasive, aggressive pathogen or group of pathogens striving towards a common goal of survival and thriving. Following the above, apperceiving not a community but an organism (see Chapter 6) is a short leap; not of faith, but of perspective.

Interventions other than issuing micromolecular drugs lag behind in use under guidance by (some) genetic component of the patient. Such cases include, but are not restricted to, radiotherapy, immunotherapy and vaccination. Various profiles are expected, ranging from tolerance and lack of efficacy to very violent adverse reactions to immunotherapy and radiotherapy (Patel and Khan 2017, Johnson et al. 2019). But vaccines are the most backward, with doses being standard for almost the entire population, at least adult, which remains a very questionable proposition. Numerous profiles of immune responses to vaccination are also expected and would range from impotence to very violent reactions.

In the context of optimization of interventions as described above, dosage should be considered as a universal factor of individualization of diverse therapies, informed mainly but not exclusively by applicable body-mass indices and, subsequently, upon detection and validation by genomic indices. The dynamics and kinetics in many cases are unknown in detail, especially their genomic background, but this is not a good reason for not tackling the issue and ignoring it in successive generations—and guidelines—of preparations. It would rather be a motive to press on, by diverse and various means, including but not limited to wet simulations, into generating relevant data, as occurred with pharmacogenomics and now pays dividends handsomely (Tsermpini et al. 2014, 2020). As biopharmaceuticals may not apply to conventional liquid and dry dosage units as used for micromolecular compounds, there is a need to establish dosage metrics for all biopharmaceuticals and find bioequivalences for very different products and thus for different dosage metrics. The use of proteins and non-protein toxins and bioregulators (not to even mention cells or phages) cannot be comparatively described by mass or volume metrics, for peptides may vary amongst themselves in terms of size and much more so in cases when there is a peptide and a non-peptide molecule or microorganism of competing preparations (bioequivalent) with the same biological action without implementing the same mechanism.

A matter of balance: To drug or not to drug?

The notion of the germ-ganism would manifest itself in therapeutics in three main ways: (i) by hacking its communication protocols, an infection may be stopped altogether or become more manageable if pseudo-signals are effected to pause pathogen propagation and/or toxin production; (ii) by introducing select microbiota, the synthesis and attitude of the germ-ganism may change and become less aggressive (or more competitive, in some occasions, as in fielding it against another threat entity); (iii) by using one or more germ-ganisms against other threats like tumors and other germ-ganisms.

The abovementioned prospective applications of the germ-ganism are based on two suppositions. The first is that the growth of a germ population may be checked and kept steady at a given set of conditions, meaning there is a set population size that is to be attained before the colony or germ-ganism stops growth and reverts to maintenance and homeostasis. This, in turn, implies (but does not guarantee) different growth maxima of such a population, in different conditions. We lack universal conclusions, but there must be some tolerance for the size of a population in different sets of environmental conditions. If environmental deterioration exceeds some threshold set rather in an effects-based manner, different and lower population maxima would be allowed, as with human body size under conditions of starvation versus adequacy of foodstuff. It follows that if the population is left to establish itself by reaching its critical size, growth will stop. If not, for example when immune responses and/or antimicrobial compounds exterminate numerous cells of the germ-ganism, the collective growth will continue in an attempt to implement the prescribed size, an effort that may exhaust the community/germ-ganism as well as the host's defenses, and create residual (endo-)toxins. This is obviously a very unsustainable way to combat infection; yet, this is all we have got up to this point. Slight methodological refinements achieved so far focus on the way of exterminating some germs (as in using such or other drug or antimicrobial amenity), and not on which kinds/species of germs are targeted for suppression or elimination and how their whole population(s) may be neutralized, by becoming functionally/metabolically inactivated, at least partially.

The second supposition is more appealing, as insinuated above—combined OMICS centered on transcriptomics might reveal the biochemical (or other) identity of the signaling process for 'go/stop growth' binary directives and the genetic logic circuitry involved. For such an endeavor, proper sampling would include collection from different colonies, conditions and colony sites for assessing both spatial and temporal parameters. By comparing full transcriptome analyses of the said samples, the genes implicated in the transition between growth and static phases can be identified, thus revealing the mechanism.

Innovative intervention and management opportunities in many fields would then follow. If the 'pause growth' signal is decoded, the stasis can be artificially induced by applying this signal exogenously, or by interfering in the pathway of the said signal. Consequently, the proliferation could stop at an early stage, despite the ongoing detrimental effects of the antimicrobial agents (both drugs and immune responses). This would produce an excellent enhancer agent for combatting infection and a similar prospect to contain aggressive tumors. Even feeble immune systems would be able to clear invading populations induced to stasis, for the concomitant degradation would be minimal due to the static phase and thus reduced metabolism of the pathogen, while the eliminated pathogenic cells are not replaced, at least not fast enough. This is the quintessence of the hacking approach mentioned above, although other non-medical applications could well follow. One such application would be to keep the growth steady so as to maximize metabolite production or to antagonize other germ-ganisms or threatening organisms like pests plaguing intense agricultural exploitations.

The germ-ganism transcends the whole network of infection-related functions of the host and the symbiont; in this case, the term symbiont is used inclusively/ *sensu lato* rather than strictly/*sensu stricto*; thus, it includes pathogenic symbionts/ pathobionts (de Oliveira et al. 2017). A first level of interactions involves the appendage microbiomes, as mentioned before, including but not limited to pathobiomes. The second level is the ramifications on therapies and generally of containment practices, both spontaneous (immune systems of different capabilities and principles—adaptive versus innate—in different organisms, such as plants, animals, unicellular organisms) and perpetrated (therapeutic interventions). This aspect has been discussed briefly above. The third and perhaps the most intriguing level is the prospect of therapeutic intervention by biopharmaceuticals that are based on live agents amenable to manipulations at the level of the germ-ganism. As already mentioned in this case, in industrial applications for instance, the germ-ganism handling would be tailored to increase selected growth metrics (which ones depends on the application), not suppress growth, like when tackling a pathobiome.

The deregulation of appendage microbiomes should also be considered within the therapeutic solution projected by the idea of the germ-ganism or any other integrative theory suggesting multicellular potential for generally unicellular organisms. The association is direct and not indirect. Many infectious diseases occur due to microbiome deregulation, meaning a compromise of the balance stricken between the living environment-host and the local microbiome, (a part of) which starts propagating intensely and aggressively. This change can be understood as a failure in the established homeostasis and causes a drift in normative terms (Kourilsky 2016), thus reappraising (parts of) the microbiome to alien or hostile status. The above could be well explained by the concept of the germ-ganism; the self-restrain quota, as applicable in a certain environment, do not apply any longer due to either of the two following cases, or their combination to any degree. The first case is the lifting (due to any reason, the change of the chemical environment included) of the quorum-sensing or other arrest-growth signals, which would lead some of the constituents of the microbiome into an explosive (exponential) growth phase anew. The second case refers to the change in environmental conditions that apply to some different arrest-growth patterns, more permissive, and thus initiating *de novo* explosive growth. The latter would irritate the host directly (by encroaching into the host tissues for nutrients) and indirectly (through metabolic and other byproducts). As a result, the new condition would elicit host response towards antimicrobial action to curtail such increased rate of injury (an immune response, *sensu lato*), which would in turn further explosive growth of the germ-ganism as it appreciates itself under environmental pressure at the very least.

A change of environment, for instance due to the excretions of the skin or the content of the gastro-intestinal tract due to medication or (a change in) dietary habits, is enough for such occurrences. The drastic depletion of a subpopulation of the microbiome, due to a similar event, especially the (side effects of the) administration of an antibiotic, allows room for expansion to other subpopulations of the microbiome, as is the current theory, which may be more aggressive. But, under the concept of the germ-ganism, these other subpopulations are prompted to occupy the vacuum so as to replace the biomass lost from the detrimental event—the host's immune response, irrespective its exact nature. The pattern described above refers to one appendage microbiome changing its attitude without a change in its composition. The converse is true as a new microbiote migrating into the microbiome does not just change the latter's constitution and balance, as apperceived originally. It transforms the germ-ganism into something different, another germ-ganism altogether. This 'mutated' germ-ganism (the change of the collective genome makes the term 'mutated' acceptable) would be defined by different priorities, limits and decision loops to adapt to the environment, even if the latter remains the same.

Fighting fire with fire: The biologicals

The biologicals, or biopharmaceuticals, plus their biosimilars (synthetic compounds which are almost identical in structure and function to a given biopharmaceutical) are the greatest hope against many ailments, including infectious diseases. The latter are actually prime candidates for such treatments, as there seems to be a chronic shortage of antibiotic development and production for a variety of reasons (Kambouris et al. 2017). Except for the issue of deficiencies in antibiotics development, the biopharmaceuticals may prove more sustainable in the long run, with lower environmental footprint, requiring less elaborate production facilities and thus easing the transportation burden inherent to centralized processes and the respective regulation/control tails that increase the operational costs and, ultimately, provide a much more flexible tool—or at least principle—for medical and non-medical intervention. The biopharmaceuticals where the agent fulfil cellular-level functions are also called pharmabiotics (Adhya et al. 2014). Non-pharmabiotic biopharmaceuticals are of molecular nature, including but not limited to enzymes (that may degrade toxins and viral elements), biotoxins (that may neutralize or compromise the infecting cells), bioregulators (that may uprate immune responses or degrade the physiology of the infection) and perhaps ribozymes as well.

Some examples of antimicrobial biologicals include but are not limited to the following: (i) viruses and phages engineered to attack specifically tumor cells (oncolytic viruses-virotherapy, see below) and possibly bacteria (bacteriophages), with an increased and perhaps programmable affinity for such cells; (ii) bacteriophages selected to take out specific bacteria in a bacteriome and virophages to combat viral infections; (iii) cells (bacteria/fungi) endowed with the ability to produce moderately powerful and fast-degradable toxins that would present minimum diffusion into the healthy tissues and blood dispersion into other body compartments. Such toxins should show affinity for some pathogen, internal (autopathogens) or invading, and low cross-reactivity/affinity towards healthy host cells; and (iv) vectors—including but not restricted to viral ones—conferring such abilities to the host cells, especially in non-medical settings.

These are only the more obvious of the possible aspects of using microbiomics to treat tumors and infections. In the latter case, a biotoxin would be intended for countering infection by degrading the infectious agents or alleviating a cytokine storm (Debnath et al. 2020, Hu et al. 2021). An inductive bioregulator would promote healing (partially or wholly) to undo a deregulation ailment, including but not limited to psychiatric conditions. Of course, any other conceivable amenity, such as nutrients or enzymes, could be the direct effector.

Beyond that, and irrespective of whether there is a biosecurity aspect to be sought, other cases would also be applicable. These may include the conditioning or perhaps even engineering of the microbiome so as to forestall, relieve or even heal autoimmune ailments. The regulation of different aspects of signaling by a more balanced function of the gut-brain axis, possibly helping mental conditions and definitely contributing to endocrinopathies (Lee and Abizaid 2014, Johnson and Foster 2018), would be less complicated and demanding.

Viruses, if taken as forms of life, should have a domain of their own (Desnues et al. 2012): the Akarya, wherein viroids would also be included. According to whether they are considered forms of life or not, they are included under the pharmabiotics or the biopharmaceuticals respectively. Their use can be identified in many levels, the obvious one being that of effectors, as in cancer virotherapy (Nettelbeck et al. 2021). A less obvious one is as probes, wherein their high affinity and specificity for their targets allows accurate delivery of signaling or destructive moieties. In the case of phages, their narrow bacterial host range guarantees limited probability for perturbations to host eukaryotic cells and attachment to benign microbiota (Adhya et al. 2014) while delivering to their targets either identification molecules, such as dyes, chromophores, radiophores or other tags (Awasthi et al. 2004, Liu et al. 2020) or highly lethal but not very specific effectors. Such effectors include radiomoieties (NCI Staff 2020), therapeutic or toxic proteins and other toxins (Kontermann et al. 2021, Nettelbeck et al. 2021) or amplification particles, the paradigm being that of gold nanoparticles for photothermal cancer therapy (Ahmad et al. 2016, Vines et al. 2019), which amplify specific wavelengths locally to cause intense thermal damage to spatially strictly defined and localized tumor cells.

The employment of native or naturally occurring, biotechnologically modified or totally engineered viruses as effectors to infect and incapacitate/lyse target cells (Kaufman et al. 2015), potentially in many quantitatively expanding infectious cycles refers mostly (but by no means exclusively) to the use of phages against bacteria. The sector is thriving with combination therapies of phages and antibiotics not only tried but studied to the degree of establishing the Phage-Antibiotics Synergy (PAS) effect (Li et al. 2021). Although there are viruses for every form of life, including fungi and protozoan parasites (Sutela et al. 2019, Barrow et al. 2020), few direct applications other than bacteriophages seem to draw attention (Barrow et al. 2020). The Virophages may be of interest (Taylor et al. 2014, Dutta et al. 2021), along with oncolytic viruses, with high affinity against cancerous cells (Kaufman et al. 2015, Kontermann et al. 2021). In all these cases, the phenomenon of viral interference should be exploited to maximize effectiveness against respective targets (Adhya et al. 2014).

Viral interference keeps already infected cells secure from additional viral infections (Dianzani 1975, Escobedo-Bonilla 2021). It should be examined on a case-to-case basis whether a self-imposed limitation accounts for the minimization of multiple and perhaps combined cellular infections rather than a preventive mechanism of the host population like interferon, which got its name from this very phenomenon (Dianzani 1975). There are prospects hiding in this pattern, which are more interesting than the optimization of the infective potential of a given population of virions. For example, less threatening viral infections caused intentionally by treating a patient proactively or reactively with low-impact viral strains may disrupt the infectious cycle of more virulent and pathogenic species and strains, making epidemics die out due to antagonism. A step further would be to use interference to ward off viral infections altogether. By mimicking the docking signal of the host cells, through some surface signal or tag, live virions would be discouraged to dock and infect, and consequently the number of infected cells would be kept low, thus thwarting the onset of disease enough for other intervention approaches to take effect, or the immune response of the host to come up to speed.

In a different setting, therapeutic biotoxins (Foster 2009), perhaps wholly designed and developed *in vitro*, but encoded in engineered vectors, would offer a mechanistic alternative to delivery by injection and *per os*. This approach would allow better regulated and adaptable release by the vector and, most importantly, the *in situ* synthesis of the effector agent, thus making away with many biosafety issues inherent to delivery pathways. This of course applies as long as the vector can be targeted exclusively to the biosite of interest.

If a small inoculum of a pharmabiotics agent is administered, it would take some time to establish itself into its intended habitat, to overcome ecological difficulties and reach the expected size. There are many issues that require elucidation and modeling. An erroneously calculated inoculum size would be very risky, for it could bring about the expected results and then nullify them by the pharmabiotic agent reaching itself the proportions of an infection and its septic/toxic reverse effects. If some detrimental population (like surging infectious cells or explosively growing tumors) are to be countered, an inoculum small enough, to be aggressively attacking and feeding on such encroachers, but large enough to allow readily measurable results and to securely establish itself, should be considered.

And this is where the germ-ganism comes into play. The introduction/transfer of a fully-fledged germ-gansim at the site of interest would mean that the desired effects set in early, these being for example an antagonistic/hostile/predatory relation with the target cell population, or the production of a metabolite.

Similarly, by using a viral biopharmaceutical against a cellular infectious disease (or a viral one, actually), the swarming kinetics would multiply both safety and efficacy: smaller numbers of administered virions would suffice to engage a number to target entities, either solely to neutralize them or to neutralize them and propagate to continue with successive circles of cell lysis and thus depleting the targeted population. The number of administered virions kept to a minimum diminishes the risk of collateral damage to healthy tissues by abundance of uncommitted virions and also of virus mutation towards strains either injurious to the host or simply ineffective ones.

Biocybernetics: Fiction of today, fact of tomorrow or a concept of the past?

The main idea behind biocybernetics, a decades-old term, is the application of control systems, technology and principles to biological entities. The original was focused obviously on the realm of the nervous system on one hand and of the complex regulation of homeostasis on the other (Red'ko 1998, Goldstein and Kopin 2017). The overhauled and revamped idea, though, rather suggests the exercise of controlling bioentities, especially organisms of any size, by executive orders through biological signaling and not through conventional training which may be inapplicable; also, the commanding authority is understood to be intelligent in nature and xenobiotic towards the subject.

The germ-ganism meets the field of biocybernetics in all the cases where a manipulator would try to tamper with the control and signaling processes of the germ-ganism or with the respective authorities/centers (rough analogues to the brain). The biocybernetics approach has been mentioned above as, in theory, it allows considerable leverage compared to the usual processes based on direct effectors, the toxin-antitoxin gene pairs for example (Hammer 2018), in any creative format and application. Biocybernetics may resolve infections, for they do not center the response around cellular effectors which lead to (i) an exchange of cellular damage and the production of toxic waste and metabolites and (ii) self-endangering responses (mostly through cytokines and chemokines) including but not limited to allergy and inflammation (Cribbs et al. 2020). The basic application in resolving infections of any host and also contamination of non-living substrates (like microbial degradation of artefacts and resources) is the crudest application of biocybernetics. It bridges well with new concepts in military science, inspired conceptually and procedurally by biological processes (Kourilsky 2016, O'Donoughue et al. 2021, Unknown 2018). By delivering very limited quantities of some (not necessarily biochemical) agent for which the offending cells do not possess resistance or counters, for it is autologous, a "friendlie" in military parlance-or, more accurately, an autobiotic—the same functional effect is reached. This is the arrest of growth and perhaps of development as well, without the mayhem and damage caused by the massive intervention of the immune system or of antiseptics, antibiotics and other destructive amenities.

The next step is to identify signals that induce hibernation and any other kind of stasis so as to pause the production of biotoxins, may these be main products or metabolic byproducts. Similarly, the other direction of this, the second step of research, is the possible identification in different microbial taxa of the functional analogue of apoptotic signals; this is actually microbial Programmed Cell Death (PCD) which has attracted the interest of researchers lately (Hammer 2018). At least in eykaryotic pathogens, one would attempt to guess that similar entities are included in the genomic blueprint and did not appear evolutionarily *de novo* in multicellular, highly differentiated macroorganisms; although, the latter may not be true since such integrated negatively regulating procedures may well be one of the secrets that allowed the higher evolution of the affected species.

The idea described above may evolve in different levels, one being the nature of signals. EM signals can be applicable, directly or by interfering with the proper, standard signaling mechanism by any conceivable chain of effects (Siamoglou et al. 2020). The extreme progress in EM transmission technology would allow faster breakthroughs in many different levels once the course is validated as potentially effective, although issues of reproducibility and applicability in diverse environments with different EM compatibility peculiarities must be addressed and resolved. Mechanical stimuli, being interpretable as signals such as pressure waves or simple application of pressure, may be exploited as well.

Another level is, of course, the inductive application, as to how tampering with the signaling process might stimulate the cells to a desired mode of growing: (a) growing fast which means accelerated metabolism and higher efficiency in desired biochemical reactions, as when using microorganisms to decompose waste, (b) growing faster but, more importantly, for more generations than their ontogenetic blueprint specifies for a given set of conditions in order to produce more biomass, or (c) growing directionally to enrich a substrate or decontaminate another. Alternatively, (d) they may be "persuaded" to remain steady in population size (or cellular size for that matter) so as to maximize the production of metabolites, a key issue in agriculture, health and in some industries (of various sizes) engaging in the production of minimally processed or bioprocessed foods and beverages; other applications of similar nature also exist: drugs (antibiotics included) and essences (preservatives included) for instance.

The ultimate stage of development of biocybernetics is to integrate or disintegrate germ-ganism(s). The obvious objective is to manipulate different germ-ganisms to antagonize or to cooperate, depending upon the context. The context of antagonism is highly suited to the prevention of infection from occurring or progressing, or to reduce the extent of contamination. A cooperative mode would allow temporally and qualitatively better and quantitatively more efficient shaping of environments, such as soil enrichment, bioreclamation or bioremediation of wastelands due to organic pollutants, surface mining and terraforming processes, for colonization on earth or beyond, etc.

However, the possibility of dissolving the loose association of a germ-ganism into several parts, each of which is prone to assume germ-ganism characteristics, and then prompting these to antagonize or pray at each other is an even more intriguing prospect. The idea in principle is similar to the creation of identical twins (by splitting the early spawn of the zygote) and is validated when collecting inocula of multicellular organisms under strict regulation, which, upon transfer to benign and supportive environments, start propagating anew, beyond their developmental programming at the site of sampling. Thus, a mycelial sample may grow on a fresh petri dish even when the surrounding tissue does not heal the wound or replenish the collected tissue (Kambouris et al. 2022). A rather cohesive germ-ganism under stasis by regulation thus re-enters developmental phases. Tree branches competently cut (stem cuts) may also develop roots and give birth to new trees even when the branch has no rhizoids. It is a matter of stem cells in multicellular organisms and, obviously, of regulation in colonial unicellular ones. By dividing a microbiome or a germ-ganism (like a biofilm) into multiple parts, possibly in spatially dispersed enclaves communicating by distance amenities, ecological friction may be caused which, in its turn, may be incensing antagonism and/or the production of some metabolites and the assumption of specific forms.

The production of the said metabolites (pure in the case of homogeneous sub-germ-ganisms, mixed in polymicrobial/chimeric ones) may be used in infection/disinfection/decon applications, antineoplastic or immunosuppressive regimens, and anti-inflammatory and regulatory therapies (including the treatment of autoimmune syndromes). The development of a specific form and phenotype would, on the other hand, allow for more accurate identification, evolving the principle of growing (micro) organisms on restrictive substrates to develop highly characteristic phenotypes (may these be morphological characters/morphophenotypes or functional phenotypes/ergophenotypes or both), the case of mycelial fungi grown in CzA being one such example.

References

Adhya, S. et al. (2014). Therapeutic and prophylactic applications of bacteriophage components in modern medicine.Cold Spring Harbor Perspectives in Medicine, 4(1). doi: 10.1101/cshperspect.a012518.

Ahmad, R. et al. (2016). Advanced gold nanomaterials for photothermal therapy of cancer. Journal of Nanoscience and Nanotechnology, 16(1): 67–80. doi: 10.1166/JNN.2016.10770.

Awasthi, V. et al. (2004). Biodistribution of radioiodinated adenovirus fiber protein knob domain after intravenous injection in mice. Journal of Virology, 78(12): 6431–6438. doi: 10.1128/JVI.78.12.6431-6438.2004.

Barrow, P. et al. (2020). Viruses of protozoan parasites and viral therapy: Is the time now right? Virology Journal, 17(1). doi: 10.1186/S12985-020-01410-1.

Benninger, F. and Steiner, I. (2018). CSF in acute and chronic infectious diseases. Handbook of Clinical Neurology, 146: 187. doi: 10.1016/B978-0-12-804279-3.00012-5.

Cribbs, S.K. et al. (2020). Pathogenesis of HIV-related lung disease: Immunity, infection, and inflammation. Physiological Reviews, 100(2): 603–632. doi: 10.1152/PHYSREV.00039.2018.

Debnath, M. et al. (2020). Genetic gateways to COVID-19 infection: Implications for risk, severity, and outcomes. FASEB Journal, 34(7): 8787–8795. doi: 10.1096/fj.202001115R.

Declerck, P.J. (2012). Biologicals and biosimilars: A review of the science and its implications. Generics and Biosimilars Initiative Journal, 1(1): 13–16. doi: 10.5639/gabij.2012.0101.005.

Desnues, C., Boyer, M. and Raoult, D. (2012). Sputnik, a Virophage Infecting the Viral Domain of Life. Advances in Virus Research, 82: 63–89. doi: 10.1016/B978-0-12-394621-8.00013-3.

Dianzani, F. (1975). Viral interference and interferon. La Ricerca in Clinica e in Laboratorio, 5(3): 196–213. doi: 10.1007/BF02908284.

Dutta, D. et al. (2021). Virophages: Association with human diseases and their predicted role as virus killers. Pathogens and Disease, 79(8). doi: 10.1093/FEMSPD/FTAB049.

Escobedo-Bonilla, C.M. (2021). Mini review: Virus interference: history, types and occurrence in Crustaceans. Frontiers in Immunology, 12: 2332. doi: 10.3389/FIMMU.2021.674216/BIBTEX.

Foster, K.A. (2009). Engineered toxins: New therapeutics. Toxicon, 54(5): 587–592. doi: 10.1016/J.TOXICON.2009.01.037.

Goldstein, D.S. and Kopin, I.J. (2017). Homeostatic systems, biocybernetics, and autonomic neuroscience. Autonomic Neuroscience : Basic & Clinical, 208: 15–28. doi: 10.1016/J.AUTNEU.2017.09.001.

Hammer, N.D. (2018). Microbial programmed cell death. Apoptosis and Beyond: The Many Ways Cells Die. John Wiley & Sons, Ltd, pp. 49–70. doi: 10.1002/9781119432463.CH3.

Hu, B. et al. (2021). The cytokine storm and COVID-19. Journal of Medical Virology, 93(1): 250–256. doi: 10.1002/JMV.26232.

Johnson, K. et al. (2019). Genetic variants predict optimal timing of radiotherapy to reduce side-effects in breast cancer patients. Clinical Oncology, 31(1): 9–16. doi: 10.1016/J.CLON.2018.10.001.

Johnson, K.V.-A. and Foster, K.R. (2018). Why does the microbiome affect behaviour? Nature Reviews Microbiology, 16(10): 647–655. doi: 10.1038/s41579-018-0014-3.

Kambouris, M.E. (2017). Wireless electrostimulation: A new approach in combating infection? Future Microbiology, 12(3): 255–65. doi: 10.2217/fmb-2017-0157.

Kambouris, M.E. et al. (2018). Rebooting Bioresilience: A Multi-OMICS approach to tackle global catastrophic biological risks and next-generation biothreats. OMICS A Journal of Integrative Biology, 22(1): 35–51. doi: 10.1089/omi.2017.0185.

Kambouris, M.E. et al. (2021). The emerging pathogens: Nature, status, and threat. In Genomics in Biosecurity. 1st edn. London: Elsevier Academic Press, pp. 61–74.

Kambouris, M.E. et al. (2022). Beyond the microbiome: germ-ganism? An integrative idea for microbial existence, organization, growth, pathogenicity, and therapeutics. Omics : A Journal of Integrative Biology, 26(4): 204–217. doi: 10.1089/OMI.2022.0015.

Kaminskaia, N.V. et al. (2000). Hydrolysis of β-lactam antibiotics catalyzed by dinuclear zinc(II) complexes: Functional mimics of metallo-β-lactamases. Journal of the American Chemical Society, 122(27): 6411–6422. doi: 10.1021/JA993704L/SUPPL_FILE/JA993704L_SA.PDF.

Karavitis, J. and Kovacs, E. (2011). Macrophage phagocytosis: Effects of environmental pollutants, alcohol, cigarette smoke, and other external factors. J Leukoc Biol, 90(6): 1065–78. doi: 10.1189/jlb.0311114.

Kaufman, H.L. et al. (2015). Oncolytic viruses: A new class of immunotherapy drugs. Nature Reviews. Drug Discovery, 14(9): 642. doi: 10.1038/NRD4663.

Kontermann, R.E. et al. (2021). Viro-antibody therapy: Engineering oncolytic viruses for genetic delivery of diverse antibody-based biotherapeutics. mAbs, 13(1). doi: 10.1080/19420862.2021.1982447.

Kourilsky, P. (2016). The natural defense system and the normative self model. F1000Research, 5: 797. doi: 10.12688/F1000RESEARCH.8518.1/DOI.

Lang, M. et al. (2020). Non-surgical treatment options for pulmonary aspergilloma. Respiratory Medicine, 164. doi: 10.1016/j.rmed.2020.105903.

Lee, C.Y. and Abizaid, A. (2014). The gut–brain-axis as a target to treat stress-induced obesity. Frontiers in Endocrinology, 5: 117. doi: 10.3389/FENDO.2014.00117.

Li, X. et al. (2021). A combination therapy of Phages and Antibiotics: Two is better than one. International Journal of Biological Sciences, 17(13): 3573. doi: 10.7150/IJBS.60551.

Liu, F. et al. (2020). Construction of eGFP-tagged senecavirus a for facilitating virus neutralization test and antiviral assay. Viruses. Viruses, 12(3). doi: 10.3390/V12030283.

NCI Staff. (2020). Radiopharmaceuticals Emerging as New Cancer Therapy - NCI, National Cancer Institute. Available at: https://www.cancer.gov/news-events/cancer-currents-blog/2020/radiopharmaceuticals-cancer-radiation-therapy (Accessed: 20 August 2022).

Nettelbeck, D.M. et al. (2021). Virotherapy in Germany—Recent Activities in Virus Engineering, Preclinical Development, and Clinical Studies. Viruses. Multidisciplinary Digital Publishing Institute (MDPI), 13(8). doi: 10.3390/V13081420.

O'Donoughue, N. et al. (2021). Distributed kill chainsNo Title. Santa Monica.

de Oliveira, G.L.V. et al. (2017). Intestinal dysbiosis and probiotic applications in autoimmune diseases. Immunology, 152(1): 1–12. doi: 10.1111/imm.12765.

Patel, S.V. and Khan, D.A. (2017). Adverse reactions to biologic therapy. Immunology and Allergy Clinics of North America. Immunol Allergy Clin North Am, 37(2): 397–412. doi: 10.1016/J. IAC.2017.01.012.

Red'ko, V. (1998). Problema proiskhozhdeniia intellekta i évoliutsionnaia biokibernetika [The problem of the origin of intellect and evolutionary biocybernetics]. Zh Vyssh Nerv Deiat Im I P Pavlova, 48(2): 358–69.

Schrettl, M. and Haas, H. (2011). 'Iron homeostasis—Achilles' heel of Aspergillus fumigatus? Current Opinion in Microbiology. Elsevier, 14(4): 400. doi: 10.1016/J.MIB.2011.06.002.

Siamoglou, S. et al. (2020). Electromagnetism and the microbiome(s). pp. 299–331. *In:* Kambouris, M.E. and Velegraki, A. (eds.). Microbiomics: Dimensions, Applications, and Translational Implications of Human and Environmental Microbiome Research. ELSEVIER ACADEMIC PRESS.

Sutela, S. et al. (2019). Viruses of fungi and oomycetes in the soil environment. FEMS microbiology ecology. FEMS Microbiol Ecol, 95(9). doi: 10.1093/FEMSEC/FIZ119.

Taylor, B.P. et al. (2014). The virus of my virus is my friend: Ecological effects of virophage with alternative modes of coinfection. Journal of Theoretical Biology. Academic Press, 354: 124–136. doi: 10.1016/j.jtbi.2014.03.008.

Tsermpini, E. et al. (2014). Individualizing clozapine and risperidone treatment for schizophrenia patients. Pharmacogenomics. Pharmacogenomics, 15(1): 95–110. doi: 10.2217/PGS.13.219.

Tsermpini, E.E. et al. (2020). Clinical implementation of preemptive pharmacogenomics in psychiatry: The "PREPARE" study. Psychiatrike = Psychiatriki. Greece, 31(4): 341–351. doi: 10.22365/jpsych.2020.314.341.

Unknown. (2018). Biodefense in the Age of Synthetic Biology. National Academies of Sciences, Engineering, and Medicine—NASEM 11, Washington, DC: The National Academies Press.

Vines, J.B. et al. (2019). Gold Nanoparticles for Photothermal Cancer Therapy. Frontiers in Chemistry. Frontiers Media SA, 7(APR). doi: 10.3389/FCHEM.2019.00167.

8

Cyberbiosecurity
The Threat of the Sages

Ioannis Chatzis,[1,*] *Periklis Rompolas,*[2]
Christoforos Karachristos[3] and *Angeliki Grivopoulou*[4]

Introduction

Cyberbiosecurity is an emerging field in which Cybersecurity and Biosecurity (Millett et al. 2019), along with the physical aspects of cybersecurity that relate to biological systems, are combined (Albert et al. 2021, Aruru et al. 2021). It aims at identifying and mitigating security risks amplified by the digitization of biology and automation of biotechnology. In particular, cyberbiosecurity examines the strategic use of cyberspace as a source of information flow and extraction in order to effectively support and implement biosecurity policies. Basically, cyberbiosecurity is a part of a system of measures that collectively aim to "safeguard the bioeconomy" in its broader sense—a goal described by the National Academies of Sciences, Engineering and Medicine of the United States of America (Potter et al. 2021). Based on the existing expertise and the current state of the bioeconomy, there are various causal aspects as a function of its unique characteristics that may cause unintentional or intentional harm to the human health or to the environment, with dimensions related to public health or national security in general.

Moreover, in recent years, development in networking and cooperation between public and private sector stakeholders has allowed the creation of network

[1] Public Institute of Vocational Training of Messolonghi, Messolonghi, Greece.
[2] Department of Nursing, Cyprus University of Technology, Limassol, Cyprus.
  Email: periklis_robolas@yahoo.gr
[3] Hellenic Open University, Patras, Greece.
  Email: karachrist@eap.gr
[4] Second Chance School of Messolonghi, Messolonghi, Greece.
  Email: agrivopoulou@gmail.com
* Corresponding author: yhatzis@gmail.com

infrastructures that are specifically adapted to the needs of different applications intended for data networks. At the same time, within this framework, the creation of favorable environments for the development and evaluation of new architectures of data networks and protocols can be supported (George 2019, Schabacker et al. 2019). The sharing of technological infrastructures, such as routing devices and communication channels, leads to concerns associated with the security of transmitted data, despite the widespread application of such practices. Thus, it is necessary to provide protection to the infrastructures of these networks for enabling their use in truly large-scale applications (Bays et al. 2015) (like the communication of health and clinical information at a large-population level), especially in an executable form. Cyberbiosecurity is now a new sub-field of global biosecurity, with a key goal of exploring the ever-increasing interdependence of cyberspace and biosecurity.

Cyberbiosecurity threats and challenges

Cyberbiosecurity threats are becoming increasingly important in the modern world as exceptional technological progress occurs, at a steadily accelerating pace, especially in areas such as artificial intelligence (AI) and automation in personalized therapy and synthetic biology. The above showcase the interface between information and communication technologies on one hand and of life sciences on the other. A typical example is a series of cyberattacks targeting companies and government agencies that were distributing coronavirus vaccines around the world, as discovered by the IBM's Cybersecurity division, although it is unclear whether the ultimate goal was to gain access to the technology while the vaccines were kept in the refrigerator during transportation, or to sabotage the proper distribution procedures (Patterson 2020, Sanger and LaFraniere 2020). Moreover, the increasing digitization of practices in biosciences creates new challenges for cybersecurity; these challenges involve understanding the evolving field of threats and identifying new risks. This translates, for instance, to the development of appropriate data security measures, their validation and implementation, and specific critical risks and consequences, particularly the ones associated with life sciences (Mueller 2021).

The interest in this specific field has increased in recent years; a significant number of studies have dealt with cyberbiosecurity issues, emphasizing the risks in the field of biotechnology, while also recommending preventive measures and protection against related threats for the new digital tools of life sciences and health sciences. This has been considered even more urgent for the provision of healthcare services through a digital horizon, telemedicine being a typical example (Albert et al. 2021). Still, although of important social footprint, telemedicine—and the digital horizon in healthcare provision is neither an exclusive area for the application of cyberbiosecurity, nor the most urgent one: other functions may be more severely affected. If not automated, the operation of response mechanisms and services is in most cases at least computerized and occasionally computer-assisted in decision processes. Tampering these functions can result in true-world chaos, like the dispatch of ambulances, intervention teams, supplies and assistance of any kind to the wrong places, actually anywhere but where they are needed and requested, and prospectively, where they may cause traffic jams and chaos. Should this occur in matters of urgency or of long range, where resources like ambulance helicopters (Figure 8.1) and airborne transporters are low in availability, mission failures will multiply and this might cause a cascading effect, especially with the failure of timely quarantine and curfews; such events can well result in a pandemic outbreak and a potential GCBR.

Challenges associated with cybersecurity threats are a cause of concern due to the potential social, economic, psychological and other adverse consequences that they may cause when affecting life sciences or biosciences (Craig Reed and Dunaway 2019). Thus, resilience is required especially in the area of typical network architectures and possible ways for exploiting their vulnerabilities by cyber attackers, through the study of exposure indicators and development of intrusion detection systems (Millett et al. 2019).

Cybersecurity when intended for a biological application has different aspects than in other cases (Mueller 2021). The expanding digitization of life sciences gives additional value to all the data generated, the information captured, gathered or mined, and the knowledge gained. The inability to protect data would affect the ability of a company or country to profitably participate in the upcoming fourth industrial revolution (Wang 2018, Mantle et al. 2019), for the increased reliance on process automation, along with sharing of large volumes of information, including but not limited to the concept of Big Data, using the Internet—including the Internet of Things (IoT), makes the related infrastructures vulnerable targets of extremely high impact (Potter et al. 2021).

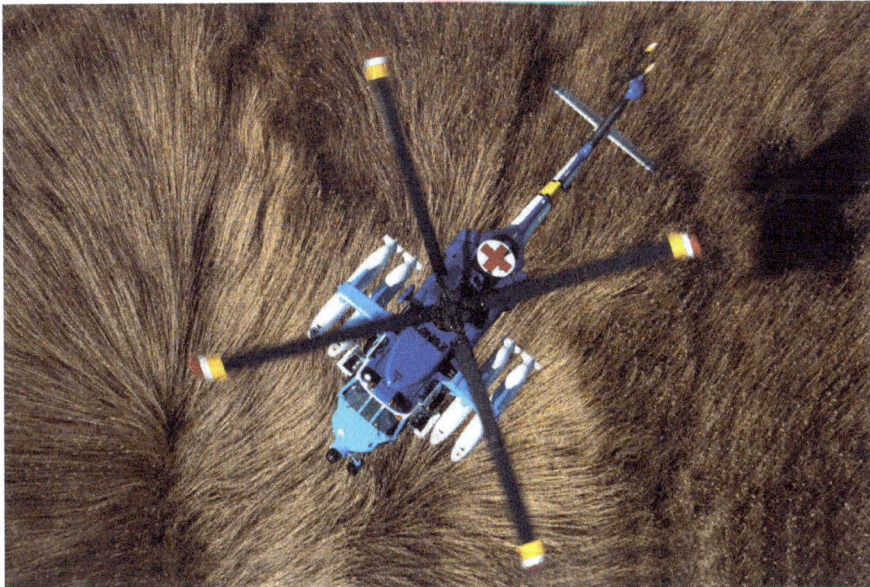

Figure 8.1. Hacking communication may divert responses, to undermine the onset of response in a timely manner. Affected operations may include inserting surveillance and test teams to establish hot zones and the nature of an incident, hauling supplies, transporting responders to and extracting casualties (medevac missions) from hot zones and even translocating subjects and objects for thorough testing and sampling, (Photo: Sikorsky Aircraft®)

Failure to safeguard these interrelated human resources and hardware and software resources against unauthorized access by third parties increases the risk of accidental or intentional damage (for example, from loss of control of any production chain or of the biosafety and quality control automation processes that pertain to the production of biological products). For instance, a laboratory information management system (LIMS) is commonly used to facilitate laboratory activities. However, current LIMS do not contain functions to improve the safety of laboratory work—the main concern of laboratories graded by biosafety levels (BSL). With loads of biosafety information to manage and a growing number of biosafety-related research projects underway, it is worth the while to expand the current LIMS framework and create a system that is more amenable for use in BSL infrastructures. Such a system should carefully balance the safety and efficiency of routine laboratory activities, allowing laboratory personnel to conduct their research as freely as possible, while ensuring the safety of the institution proper and of the environment. In order to achieve this goal, data concerning research content, laboratory personnel, experimental hardware and provisions (such as expendables, (bio)chemicals and equipment/instrumentation) must be properly stored in and fully utilized by a central system and its databases (Kolia et al. 2021, Sun et al. 2021, Wang et al. 2021). Therefore, strong cybersecurity measures are vital both for the security of data generated by the biotechnology sector and for securing the basic infrastructures and products/services they offer, that is, spanning the full spectrum of provision and production (Millett et al. 2019).

The maintenance of microbial populations of biotechnological interest at acceptable levels and the control of their toxin production in combination with their thallic or vegetative form (airborne or otherwise) are generally controlled by sophisticated environmental control systems that operate under cyber control in industry, but sometimes in academic research laboratory settings as well.

Furthermore, a successful biosecurity framework includes stakeholder participation, collaboration in troubleshooting, simplification of the definition of cyberbiosecurity, and development of a common language among experts. At the same time, awareness is needed about cybersecurity within and among the sectors of the agro food industry. Addressing the risks concerning both the pillars—agriculture and the food production industry—is not merely an IT issue, for other aspects of security are also involved (Murch et al. 2018, Peccoud et al. 2018)—especially agrosecurity/anti-agro terrorism and of course government infrastructure, all of them appearing occasionally in sophisticated forms such as precision agriculture.

Another example is a possible bioattack on urban water collection and management systems (using drones for instance), resulting in the contamination (bioterrorism) of drinking water, with the aim of spreading disease to the inhabitants of a city, while the same can happen with a cyber-attack aimed at the cleaning/processing/disinfection system of a water supply network. With a lower supply of chlorine, microbes overgrow, thus resulting in waterborne infections at epidemic levels; whereas hyperchlorination causes rather severe symptoms of chemical poisoning in the population. An important risk is also the possibility of a cyber-attack aiming to degrade the IT systems in storage areas where large batches of drugs, vaccines or equipment to deal with biological threats are kept, or to render them unsafe, resulting in enormous social, economic and political cost to a state. The paradigm in such a scenario is to tamper with the air-conditioning system to reduce cooling in the storage areas of mRNA vaccines.

Particularly in the 21st century, as the field of biodefense intersects with cyberspace, cyberthreats can have serious economic and social impact. In the field of cyberbiosecurity, the coupling of biotechnology and cybersecurity gives rise to various points of combinatorial vulnerability—an asymmetric and newly emerging critical problem for biodefense planning and consideration. New threats may emerge and propagate in ways that combine the attack profiles of biosecurity and cybersecurity concerns (Potter et al. 2021). A case in point is the malicious degradation of networks that control synthetic biological processes (automated or hybrid) which create new organisms (Organism Engineering), especially considering the xenobiological perspectives of synthetic biology and biomechanics (see Chapter 4). Malicious data falsification can create a superpathogen instead of a new, effective microorganism of legitimate applications. The latter can be a bioprocessing strain (e.g., for fermentation) and, most importantly, may constitute the main component of a biotechnological therapeutic formulation or of a biopharmaceutical therapeutic regimen, production of probiotics being a valid example here. Other examples of malicious falsification of biological data may include cases where malicious software can be used to modify actual fragments of DNA sequences within an individual's genome, through genetic analysis software (Pauwels 2021). Such malicious degradation of actual laboratory data could lead to misdiagnoses, with a direct impact on clinical decisions. Also, this kind of falsification of biological data could significantly affect the existing predictive models in functional genomics, including how complex genetic diseases are diagnosed and treated.

To determine the perceived risks at the interface between cybersecurity and biosecurity, an online pilot study ("Biosecure") was conducted from October to November 2017. It examined the views of internationally recognized leaders in the fields of biotechnology and cybersecurity. The key findings of the survey indicated that, owing to variations in threat types, targets and potential impacts, biosecurity risks in cyberspace were considered difficult to detect as they lurked in different aspects of social life. It was also shown that risks become greater as their level of complexity increases in relation to the existing, ineffective measures to deal with them (Millett et al. 2019).

Therefore, it appears that a continued effort to collaborate and interface the different fields of activity involved in these issues is necessary in order for both to develop a common language of communication—and possibly a concise terminology—and for better identification of threats and discussing possible ways, methods and practices for curtailing risks (Richardson et al. 2019, Mueller 2021). Developing appropriate strategies to proactively reduce Cybersecurity risks/vulnerability also requires a multidisciplinary approach to the relevant issues (Bays et al. 2015). In this sense, the Cybersecurity Atlas platform of the European Commission is a good practice. This platform supports knowledge management for mapping, categorizing and increasing cooperation among European cybersecurity experts in support of the European Union's digital strategy (European Commission 2022).

The cyberbiosecurity dimension of intense database use

Over the past 30 years, genomic databases in general, and that of pathogenic (micro) organisms in particular, have become an integral part of biological and biomedical research. Although genomic databases have not been cited as primary targets of cybersecurity threats, many such threats potentially apply to the genomic databases in the mid-term (Vinatzer et al. 2019).

Current biological research, including pathogen-related research projects, is increasingly dependent on public genomic databases that provide information on their genomic sequences, gene characterization (Aken et al. 2016), encoded protein sequences (Punta et al. 2012), protein interactions and metabolic networks for many organisms. Such data is critical in the design and implementation of biological experimental research.

In addition to the importance of protecting the products of research financed by public resources in general, developing means and methods of cyberbiosecurity for genomic databases is even more important—because these databases contain all the knowledge acquired by the global research community over many years on the one hand, and because of the potential impact of this knowledge on human, animal and plant health on the other. Publicly accessible genomic databases also serve as a unique resource for cybersecurity research aimed at protecting the bioeconomy (Murch et al. 2018, Peccoud et al. 2018), the value of which has been estimated to be up to 25% of the GDP in the US.

Hereditary (genetic) information naturally evolves by the reproduction of its carrier molecules within organisms. Mechanisms that naturally lead to changes in the DNA sequence include mutation, recombination, horizontal gene transfer, etc. The expression of this genomic information towards phenotype can change, depending on how an organism responds to its environment. This 'dependence on the context', including all the aspects of the system in which the genetic information exists, cannot always be predicted. The same DNA sequence may result in wildly different phenotypes depending on the neighboring DNA sequences, intramolecular and intermolecular interactions within the cell, and extracellular conditions. Thus, the impact of changes, whether introduced spontaneously (due to natural alteration) or maliciously (by tampering/engineering), is difficult to predict, detect and mitigate (Mantle et al. 2019).

Cybersecurity generally focuses on the confidentiality, integrity and availability of digital information (Jang-Jaccard and Nepal 2014) of all types, including genomic data. However, there has been no systematic study of past and prospective genomic database security breaches; still, cases of personal medical information subjected to ransomware/hostage attacks have been reported (Kruse et al. 2017). Although there is no public report of security breaches in molecular databases till date, existing cyberattack methods can easily target them in their current form.

Breach of confidentiality is an important element in cyberattacks and involves gaining access to sensitive personal information. Most public genomic databases do not contain sensitive personal information such as credit card numbers or social security numbers, yet they do contain an individual's genomic data, perhaps the most "personal" and important data of all.

Knowledge of the genome sequences of pathogenic microorganisms can lead to malicious use, a possibility that is a major biosecurity issue. Currently, many genomes of pathogenic microorganisms praying practically on all known Kingdoms of Life are registered in open access databases and available to anyone interested. A study in the early 2000s concluded that open access to pathogen genomes should be promoted (National Research Council (US) Committee on Genomics Databases for Bioterrorism Threat Agents 2004). Today, even the genome of an extremely high-risk pathogen like the smallpox virus, *Variola major*, is easily accessible at NCBI to any anonymous user. The risk increases when we consider the reduced cost of DNA synthesis technology and the advances in synthetic biology (Hudges 2017).

Furthermore, many pathogenic microorganisms may be weaponized (used as bioweapons), depending on their score on a number of criteria, like the infectious dose (the number of microorganisms or the amount of substances required to cause a disease), virulence (the ability to cause disease), transmissibility (the ease of transmission from person to person) and incubation time (the time between exposure to a biological agent and the onset of disease). All these characteristics are susceptible to tampering by modern biotechnology, and relevant knowledge (know-how included) is the key to any covert development of biological weapons (ENISA 2022).

In terms of ensuring the integrity of data stored in the databases, complex control and protection procedures do not seem to be applied in general. Many genomic databases have protocols for data quality control and manual curation, two well-proven (although crude) approaches to ensuring data integrity.

One potential risk is that of a perpetrator providing invalid data, with an incentive to steer future studies toward specific results. This kind of attack requires careful creation of database records by the perpetrator so as to maintain a valid format (similar to false Bank Pages for Internet scams). Such records contain data which is either totally fabricated or, at the very least, lacking prior acceptable experimental data generation procedures. However, verifying the validity of the data is particularly difficult and cannot be easily achieved using existing methods.

Another type of attack consists of incrementally inserting invalid records into a larger valid data set. For example, an attacker could download existing data from the database, extract a subset of the data and insert invalid data into it (replacement), possibly by abusing some edit feature of the database. In this case, detection mechanisms using probabilistic analysis may fail to find the invalid records, for only records with a clear violation of data integrity can be detected. Such attacks have been reported previously (Mo et al. 2010, Cárdenas et al. 2011, Esmalifalak et al. 2014).

Finally, reduced data availability is a potential concern for genomic databases. Primarily, their disruption can lead to the loss of productivity and research investment. For instance, if a diagnostic laboratory uses DNA sequences as a method to identify pathogens by comparison with records in a genomic database, database downtime will at least cause delays in identification. Despite the heavy investment in genomic sciences, it has been noticed that there is almost no research focused on protecting such data from cyberthreats (Vinatzer et al. 2019).

Cyberbiosecurity and the COVID-19 pandemic

Biology and biotechnology have changed dramatically in recent years, since their dependence on data digitization and process automation and the importance of their digital footprint in cyberspace have created new vulnerabilities. These refer to both the unintended consequences and the intended exploitation, and are largely underestimated (Mueller 2021). In particular, a research in the US, using the theoretical approaches to human security and biosafety, shows that, from the perspective of both the individual and the state, the COVID-19 pandemic poses a threat to global security (Albert et al. 2021, Aruru et al. 2021). In the context of the COVID-19 pandemic, research interest regarding cyber(bio)security has focused on the interactions between the physical existence of the pandemic and the events of interest in cyberspace (Potter et al. 2021), mainly due to the intensity of the effort of health authorities worldwide to coordinate and react through the massive use of digital technologies, especially on issues of awareness of development, alertness and communication for coordination and information.

The COVID-19 pandemic has promoted the digitalization of economic, social and political activities. This occurred indirectly—but not involuntarily—through the implementation of measures ostensibly enforced to contain movement and enact relative isolation to limit transmission, in particular through lockdowns and quarantines. A relevant example here is the implementation of digital governance for the state mechanism to respond to the economic, political and social pressures and effects of the pandemic, while laying the foundations for new approaches and priorities on issues of international and national security.

In addition, it became necessary to implement a network of cybersecurity policies set to protect life-science and biotechnological information and data from cyberattacks. A typical example is the cyberattack against the European Medicines Agency during the critical period of the process of voting and approving vaccines for the pandemic in order to undermine trust in the vaccines (ENISA 2022). As a result of the cyberattack, some of the documents obtained after illegal access to the system, including e-mail correspondences, were made public over the Internet, and then received by some media outlets. A careful investigation of the published material revealed that not all documents were published in their complete, original form; individual authentic emails were also collected from multiple folders, and digital mailboxes and titles were added by the perpetrators.

Digitalization due to the pandemic was, of course, not limited to financial transactions, but extended to the immediate measures to deal with and prevent cases, restore patients to health and manage the consequences in a wider context as well. One such example in the international context is the pioneering digital information map for the spread of the COVID-19 pandemic from Johns Hopkins University (Coronavirus Resource Center), which is an ever-updated source of COVID-19 data and expert guidance. This is where the available data on cases, deaths, tests, hospitalizations and vaccines are collected and analyzed to help the public, policymakers and healthcare professionals worldwide to cope with the pandemic (CRC 2022).

Also, during the COVID-19 pandemic, there were reports of increasing cyber threats to research databases and related activities such as the production of treatments, vaccines, disinfection chemicals, etc. (Potter et al. 2021). It is obvious that the alteration of vaccination databases could cause real chaos and many health losses if, for example, the vaccination certificates were canceled, or if people at high risk of transmission appeared as vaccinated and were therefore excluded from the vaccination program while they were kept, due to a digital error in the vaccination profile, active while working in close proximity with a large number of possible transmitters. Based on the fact that the vaccination certificate is a first and relatively raw form of personalized treatment or medical care that extends to the entire population of a state, very useful lessons can be learned about the possible effects and areas of vulnerability in the light of cyberbiosecurity, both against spontaneous/ accidental incidents and against deliberate challenges and threats within the wider field of personalized treatment or individualized therapy.

Cyberbiosecurity and electronic health record

eHealth refers to the tools and services based on information and communication technologies that improve the prevention, diagnosis, treatment, monitoring and management of individual and public health (COMMISSION OF THE EUROPEAN COMMUNITIES 2008). eHealth is also a priority for the European Union, a fact that is reflected in the Action Plan 2012–2020 for the development of eHealth forwarded by the EU to its member states. In this plan, there is a blueprint regarding the design, setup and implementation of the Electronic Health Record, with emphasis on cross-border services, such as the development and distribution of electronic health records and electronic prescription of patients (European Commission 2006, European Union 2019).

The applications of eHealth by several healthcare systems throughout the globe, such as the use of the Electronic Health Record, raise a number of legal, ethical and financial questions and safety issues. In particular, due to the large amount of health-related data, it is possible to make the appropriate clinical decision on a case-to-case basis (the quintessence of Individualized Therapy), and to identify and correct the occasional error of any healthcare professional in a timely manner. At the same time, the non-adoption of documented treatment protocols by health professionals can also raise legal issues in case of harm to the patient (Jamshed et al. 2015, Tsai et al. 2020). However, it must be stressed that the objective remains the adaptation of some generic blueprint of treatment to the patient. For the foreseeable future, this cannot be based on diagnostic algorithms exclusively, for the diversity in human pathophenotypes is extremely extensive and largely discontinuous as a function and therefore not precisely predictable. That is, ultimately, the doctor is necessary as a human factor who offers real individualization of diagnosis and treatment, and not only as an implementer of suggestions arising from constant means, such as algorithms and clinical instructions that tend to be somewhat rigid.

Of course, the confidentiality and security of health data are dominant issues in the context of implementation of eHealth services by healthcare systems. Today, more than ever before, health-related data is an attractive target for attackers (Bogle 2018, Healthare IT News Staff 2018). As more and more medical information and data are posted online, eHealth is becoming one of the preferred targets. The development of legal frameworks for the privacy and confidentiality of patient data and the use of electronic recording and storage standards are likely to enhance the secure exchange of data, and support to clinical decisions (Chao et al. 2013).

However, legal frameworks are by themselves insufficient. In case of malicious interventions, it is obvious that a massive change in the electronic health records of a population where individualized treatment is applied can be catastrophic. This can be done in a very large number of recordings, something easy for malware, with minor interventions or alterations of only a few, selective points or recordings (deletion of clinical signs of contraindications against a frequently prescribed drug, for instance). The above alteration will lead to the administration of incorrect treatments at a huge cost and probably massive loss of life and health, especially when therapeutic protocols and guidelines are used instead of empirical diagnoses and prescriptions. Although less destructive, another similar operation may favor a specific pharmaceutical preparation in terms of prescription, increasing the pharmaceutical cost or expense, destroying competition and possibly degrading the safety parameter and general quality of pharmacotherapy. Cybersecurity can also ensure the safe and ethically sound management of digital medical data stored in the information systems of the national Ministries of Health and in hospitals, for example, by protecting them from speculative searches by employers and insurance companies.

Cyberbiosecurity and disinformation

In modern times, there is enormous potential for the use of human genomic (and other -omic) data. When it comes to cyberbiosecurity, categories of biological information, especially medical information shared online, may provide leverage (if mismanaged) to destabilize entire societies. Therefore, the way in which the public, along with medical providers, perceives such data can lead to disinformation or misinformation (depending on the context) and acceptance of propaganda, undermining the flow of verified information to the community of healthcare professionals, as a result of which public health support would be threatened (Wallace-Wells 2020, Palmer et al. 2021).

Such propaganda, affecting research, could lead to the derailment of the supply chain and thus undermine the adequate production of biological products themselves. This can cause large-scale imbalances in the market and initiate a chain reaction that may jeopardize the management of a pandemic.

However, a further dark side to this is the possible, substantial alteration of research literature and results of clinical tests. This would result in disinformation, which could lead to false publications in scientific journals, thus delaying treatments for other conditions based on such data, or rendering them invalid. For example, mRNA vaccines, although only recently created for COVID-19, were based on data from previous vaccines (Garde and Saltzman 2020). In the future, it is possible that malicious agents will look forward to sabotaged research as a means to delay for decades or stop altogether a given development, mostly for competitive but also for other reasons.

There are also cross-effects in the case of coupling of agriculture and pharmaceutical production. For example, one can highlight cases where tobacco or cannabis plants are used to produce pharmaceutical ingredients or vaccines. Propaganda cyberattacks on the use of such agricultural technology can adversely affect both agricultural and pharmaceutical research simultaneously (Palca 2020). An example of a short-term benefit to be expected by the perpetrators is the good old leverage acquired over some market sector, but the long-term effects can be global and interdisciplinary.

Another example concerning biology is that of the perception created against vaccinations for Covid-19, where public support for the right to denial and the questioning of the validity of the projected safety and efficiency, even among healthcare professionals and the respective disciplines of the academic community, led to the global growth of an anti-vaccination movement. Fair questions arise about the institutional and other roles of social media giants in shushing or transmitting such propaganda (Iboi et al. 2020, Neergaard et al. 2020, Wilson και Wiysonge 2020).

The broader applications of cyberbiosecurity may ensure the constant control of cyber-information on issues of biosecurity and biopolitics. This can avert the disorientation of public opinion by disinformation or by failed predictions spread specifically on social media by alleged expert scientists, though of low prestige (Palmer et al. 2021)—a function that is censorship in all but name.

Furthermore, cyberbiosecurity should ensure the correct and ethical use of emerging cyber technologies, such as artificial intelligence, which is used to predict biohazard models, but also for the rapid decision-making process in the context of health crisis management (in pandemics or bioattacks, for instance) by allocating bandwidth and other virtual resources correctly, rather than allowing anarchy in times of need.

Conclusion

In conclusion, cybersecurity threats may emerge internationally, either intentionally or unintentionally. Each country, or rather political entity (with a functional definition, in this particular case, based on the existence of an independent health recording system, which can be at a local level, for example in the American States, or at the regional level, as in Europe), is called upon to act preventively for the early detection and neutralization of such threats. This should occur both individually (understood at the institutional level) and in cooperation with other countries or political entities. Cooperation is particularly important in some cases; for example, in instances where movement of people and transportation of goods become uncontrollable, as in migration and smuggling respectively, and are thus likely to cause biosecurity risks; or cases where telecommunications and cyber activity protocols create cybersecurity issues (by using common Internet access providers instead of specialized and controlled ones, for instance).

The widespread integration of 5G Internet will increase the speed and volume of information traffic globally and change the way digital information is shared, while the widespread use of artificial intelligence will dramatically change the global balance of power amongst states. At the same time, however, new digital threats will emerge from groups, states and individuals in possession of cutting-edge digital technology, who can use it for their own benefit as well as to achieve illegal purposes and/or national, sectorial or other goals.

In particular, many of the devices used throughout the biotechnology sector are portable and most of them are connected to the Internet. Challenges arise not only at the application level of research, but also during basic and pilot research, as well as on project design, product manufacturing and amenity (method or product) testing levels.

Cyberbiosecurity is a key part of the National Security Strategy, which, through intergovernmental cooperation, should have the protection of citizens from future cyberbiothreats and bio-hybrid attacks as its main objective. However, in the case of cyberattacks that are basically hybrid threats, it is impossible to safely identify the potential enemy, because of digitization, which functionally suspends state borders. States must now very seriously take into account the new digital risks and implement appropriate cyber policies in order to protect their critical infrastructure and national security, not only in cyberspace but also in space, with the strategic use of satellites, amongst other things, in telecommunication—the physical habitat of cyberspace.

At the same time, it is necessary to strengthen the knowledge, skills and competences of different interested individuals that are to work on the intersection of cybersecurity and biosafety. Finally, direct resources should be sought and invested to further understand cybersecurity risks in the field of biotechnology in order to develop appropriate prevention and response measures.

References

Aken, B.L. et al. (2016). The Ensembl gene annotation system. Database, 2016. doi: 10.1093/database/baw093.

Albert, C. et al. (2021). Human security as biosecurity. Politics and the Life Sciences, 40(1): 83–105. doi: 10.1017/pls.2021.1.

Aruru, M. et al. (2021). Pharmacy Emergency Preparedness and Response (PEPR): A proposed framework for expanding pharmacy professionals' roles and contributions to emergency preparedness and response during the COVID-19 pandemic and beyond. Research in Social and Administrative Pharmacy, 17(1): 1967–1977. doi: 10.1016/J.SAPHARM.2020.04.002.

Bays, L.R. et al. (2015). Virtual network security: Threats, countermeasures, and challenges. Journal of Internet Services and Applications, 6(1): 1–19. doi: 10.1186/s13174-014-0015-z.

Bogle, A. (2018). Healthcare data a growing target for hackers, cybersecurity experts warn—Science—ABC News. Available at: https://www.abc.net.au/news/science/2018-04-18/healthcare-target-for-hackers-experts-warn/9663304?nw=0 (Accessed: 21 July 2022).

Cárdenas, A.A. et al. (2011). Attacks against process control systems: Risk assessment, detection, and response. In Proceedings of the 6th International Symposium on Information, Computer and Communications Security, ASIACCS 2011, pp. 355–366. doi: 10.1145/1966913.1966959.

Chao, W.C. et al. (2013). Benefits and challenges of electronic health record system on stakeholders: A qualitative study of outpatient physicians. Journal of Medical Systems, 37(4). doi: 10.1007/s10916-013-9960-5.

COMMISSION OF THE EUROPEAN COMMUNITIES. (2008). Communication from the Commission to the European Parliament, the Council, the European Economic and Social Committee and the Committee of the Regions on telemedicine for the benefit of patients, healthcare systems and society, COM(2008)689 final. Available at: https://eur-lex.europa.eu/LexUriServ/LexUriServ.do?uri=COM:2008:0689:FIN:EN:PDF (Accessed: 08 AUGUST 2022).

Craig Reed, J. and Dunaway, N. (2019). Cyberbiosecurity Implications for the Laboratory of the Future. Frontiers in Bioengineering and Biotechnology, 7: 182. doi: 10.3389/fbioe.2019.00182.

CRC. (2022). John Hopkins University. Available at: https://coronavirus.jhu.edu/map.html (Accessed: 22 July 2022).

ENISA. (2022). Annual Report on Cybersecurity Research and Innovation Needs and Priorities.

Esmalifalak, M. et al. (2014). Machine Learning in Smart Grid. IEEE Systems Journal, 11(3): 1644–1652.

European Commission. (2006). eHealth priorities and strategies in European countries : eHealth ERA report : March 2007 : towards the establishment of a European eHealth research area. Publications Office.

European Commission. (2022). European Cybersecurity Atlas. Available at: https://cybersecurity-atlas. ec.europa.eu/ (Accessed: 14 June 2022).

European Union. (2019). e-Health Network Guidelines, EU Member States and the European Commission. Bucharest. Available at: https://ec.europa.eu/health/sites/health/files/ehealth/docs/ev_20190611_ co922_en.pdf.

Garde, D. and Saltzman, J. (2020). The story of mRNA: From a Loose Idea to a Tool that may help Curb Covid. Available at: https://www.statnews.com/2020/11/10/the-story-of-mrna-how-a-once-dismissed-idea-became-a-leading- technology-in-the-covid-vaccine-race/(Accessed: 20 July 2022)

George, A.M. (2019). The national security implications of cyberbiosecurity. Frontiers in Bioengineering and Biotechnology, 7: 51. doi: 10.3389/fbioe.2019.00051.

Healthare IT News Staff (2018). Projects. Healthare IT News. Available at: https://www.healthcareitnews. com/projects /biggest-healthcare-data-breaches-2018-so-far (Accessed: 21 July 2022).

Hudges, R. (2017). Synthetic DNA: Methods and Protocol. New York: Humana Press.

Iboi, E.A. et al. (2020). Will an imperfect vaccine curtail the COVID-19 pandemic in the US? Infectious Disease Modelling, 5: 510–524. doi:10.1016/j.idm.2020.07.006.

Jamshed, N. et al. (2015). Ethical issues in electronic health records: A general overview. Perspectives in Clinical Research, 6(2): 73. doi: 10.4103/2229-3485.153997.

Jang-Jaccard, J. and Nepal, S. (2014). A survey of emerging threats in cybersecurity. Journal of Computer and System Sciences, 80(5): 973–993. doi: 10.1016/j.jcss.2014.02.005.

Kolia, K.I. et al. (2021). Team experience of nasopharyngeal samples reception, decontamination, and sorting during the COVID-19 pandemic (2020) at Institut Pasteur Côte d'Ivoire. Journal of Biosafety and Biosecurity, 3(2): 120–124. doi: 10.1016/j.jobb.2021.08.005.

Kruse, C.S. et al. (2017). Cybersecurity in healthcare: A systematic review of modern threats and trends. Technology and Health Care, 25: 1–10. doi: 10.3233/THC-161263.

Mantle, J.L. et al. (2019). Cyberbiosecurity for biopharmaceutical products. Frontiers in Bioengineering and Biotechnology, 7: 116. doi: 10.3389/fbioe.2019.00116.

Millett, K. et al. (2019). Cyberbiosecurity risk perceptions in the biotech sector. Frontiers in Bioengineering and Biotechnology, 7: 136. doi: 10.3389/fbioe.2019.00136.

Mo, Y. et al. (2010). False data injection attacks against state estimation in wireless sensor networks. In Proceedings of the IEEE Conference on Decision and Control, pp. 5967–5972. doi: 10.1109/ CDC.2010.5718158.

Mueller, S. (2021). Facing the 2020 pandemic: What does cyberbiosecurity want us to know to safeguard the future? Biosafety and Health, 3(1): 11–21. doi: 10.1016/j.bsheal.2020.09.007.

Murch, R.S. et al. (2018). Cyberbiosecurity: An emerging new discipline to help safeguard the bioeconomy. Frontiers in Bioengineering and Biotechnology, 6: 39. doi: 10.3389/fbioe.2018.00039.

National Research Council (US) Committee on Genomics Databases for Bioterrorism Threat Agents (2004). Seeking Security: Pathogens, Open Access, and Genome Databases. Washington (DC): National Academies Press.

Neergaard, L. and Fingerhut, H. (2020). AP-NORC poll: Half of Americans would get a COVID-19 vaccine. Available at: https://apnews.com/article/ap-norc-poll-us-half-want-vaccine-shots-4d98d bfc0a64d60d52ac84c3065dac55 (Accessed: 17 June 2022)

Palca, J. (2020). Tobacco Plants Contribute Key Ingredient For COVID-19 Vaccine. Available at: https:// www.npr.org/sections/health-shots/2020/10/15/923210562/tobacco-plants-contribute-key-ingredient-for- covid-19-vaccine (Accessed: 15 July 2022).

Palmer, X.-L. et al. (2021). Matters of biocybersecurity with consideration to propaganda outlets and biological agents. In European Conference on Cyber Warfare and Security, pp. 525–533. Available at: https://www.proquest.com/conference-papers-proceedings/matters-biocybersecurity-with-consideration/docview/2555180223/se-2?accountid=27828%0Ahttp://sfx-82kst-kaist.hosted.exlibrisgroup.com/kaist?url_ver=Z39.88-2004&rft_val_fmt=info:ofi/fmt:kev:mtx:journal.

Patterson, D. (2020). Hackers are attacking the COVID-19 vaccine supply chain - CBS News. CBS News. Available at: https://www.cbsnews.com/news/covid-19-vaccine-hackers-supply-chain/ (Accessed: 21 July 2022).

Pauwels, E. (2021). Cyberbiosecurity: How to protect biotechnology from adversarial AI attacks. Hybrid CoE Strategic Analysis, 26: 3–9. Available at: www.hybridcoe.fi.

Peccoud, J. et al. (2018). Cyberbiosecurity: From Naive trust to risk awareness. Trends in Biotechnology, 36(1): 4–7. doi: 10.1016/j.tibtech.2017.10.012.

Potter, L. et al. (2021). Biocybersecurity: A converging threat as an auxiliary to war. International Conference on Cyber Warfare and Security, pp. 291–298,XIV. Available at: https://www.proquest.com/conference-papers-proceedings/biocybersecurity-converging-threat-as-auxiliary/docview/2505729708/se-2?accountid=17225.

Punta, M. et al. (2012). The Pfam protein families database. Nucleic Acids Research, 40(Database issue): D290–D301. doi: 10.1093/nar/gkr1065.

Richardson, L.C. et al. (2019). Building capacity for cyberbiosecurity training. Frontiers in Bioengineering and Biotechnology, 7: 112. doi: 10.3389/fbioe.2019.00112.

Sanger, D. and LaFraniere, S. (2020). Cyberattacks Discovered on Vaccine Distribution Operations. NY Times. Available at: https://www.nytimes.com/2020/12/03/us/politics/vaccine-cyberattacks.html (Accessed: 21 July 2022).

Schabacker, D.S. et al. (2019). Assessing cyberbiosecurity vulnerabilities and infrastructure resilience. Frontiers in Bioengineering and Biotechnology, 7: 61. doi: 10.3389/fbioe.2019.00061.

Sun, D. et al. (2021). Laboratory information management system for biosafety laboratory: Safety and efficiency. Journal of Biosafety and Biosecurity, 3: 28–34.

Tsai, C.H. et al. (2020). Effects of electronic health record implementation and barriers to adoption and use: A scoping review and qualitative analysis of the content. Life, 10(12): 1–27. doi: 10.3390/life10120327.

Vinatzer, B.A. et al. (2019). Cyberbiosecurity challenges of pathogen genome databases. Frontiers in Bioengineering and Biotechnology, 7: 1–11. doi: 10.3389/fbioe.2019.00106.

Wallace-Wells, D. (2020). 'We Had the Vaccine the Whole Time', TOMORROW. Available at: https://nymag.com/intelligencer/2020/12/moderna-covid-19-vaccine-design.html (Accessed: 21 July 2022).

Wang, B. (2018). The future of manufacturing: A new perspective. Engineering, 4(5): 722–728. doi: 10.1016/j.eng.2018.07.020.

Wang, L. et al. (2021). Tianjin biosecurity guidelines for codes of conduct for scientists: Promoting responsible sciences and strengthening biosecurity governance. Journal of Biosafety and Biosecurity, 3: 82–83.

Wilson, S.L. and Wiysonge, C. (2020). Social media and vaccine hesitancy. BMJ Global Health, 5(10): 1-7. doi: 10.1136/bmjgh-2020-004206.

9

Harnessing Fields, Waves and Currents
The Realm of Mages

M.E. Kambouris

Introduction

Electromagnetic (EM) treatment of living organisms, also known in some cases as Electrostimulation (ES), has multiple applications in biosecurity, especially if the latter is taken *sensu lato*, apart from the usefulness (especially indirect) of electromagnetic amenities in diagnostics. Its use should be understood mainly as an approach to regulate the physiology of involved organisms: potential hosts, potential or active pathogens and pathogen antagonists being the main groups with profound impact on biosecurity. This range can be expanded to include rather indirect parameters making up the functional footprint of biosecurity, like availability of information, material and energy commodities.

The EM modalities can be understood as roughly belonging to four categories, three of which are fields—electric, magnetic and combined, electromagnetic. The fourth category is that of electric current, routed directly, although possibly through some interface. Consequently, this qualifies as a conductive amenity, in contrast to the inductive nature of the other three, where results are achieved by exposing the object to a field and not by actively routing energy through it (Siamoglou et al. 2020).

The operational distinction of the use of EM is much more important than the above distinction by nature and does not strictly correspond to the four categories outlined.

University of Patras, School of Health Sciences, Department of Pharmacy, Patras, Greece & The Golden Helix Foundation, London, United Kingdom.
Email: mekambouris@yahoo.com, ORCID iD: https://orcid.org/0000-0002-3205-4797

The EM allows faster treatment of injuries (electrostimulation), with less chemical and other bulky and partially unsustainable and diverse chemical compounds, as wound healing is a primary function of such modalities. This concept includes therapy of non-human and non-animal subjects and thus has applications in agriculture as well. It could be expanded to include the anti-tumor and antimicrobial activities exercised by the different elements of immune systems, as the latter are upregulated by EM treatment, but not the actual antimicrobial, and antitumor effect. It may also allow, in the guise of electrotherapy, treatment of different non-infectious ailments like cancer and other internist conditions. A very important asset in this case is that it allows conditions being treated even when transportation, conservation and detailed communication resources are compromised, which adversely effects the prescription and distribution of ordinary medicaments.

Another direct effect, similar to therapeutics but different in details and somewhat proactively applied, is that EM may allow increased yields in crops and industrial biotechnology (Efthimiadou et al. 2014, Kambouris et al. 2014, Katsenios et al. 2016, Stathoulias et al. 2020), thus alleviating shortages caused by disruptive as well as destructive effects of bioevents or other catastrophes. This is far from a biosecurity-oriented application; its benefits are obvious for proper exploitation even under ideal conditions, especially in the case of intensive exploitation. But the increase in yield, which could be applicable to land reclamation and exploitation of barren or unfertile soil, without the use of chemical fertilizers that have huge environmental footprints and are dependent on supply chains, is instrumental in safeguarding self-sufficiency (of energy as well, by intense production of biofuel). In this way the disruptive and—to an extent—the destructive damage caused by bioevents may be curtailed. The disruptive damage is exemplified by the breaking down of transportation, mainly but not exclusively for purposes of isolation/quarantine. On the other hand, the destructive damage is amplified by the dissemination by fomites and negating the said dissemination limits the extent and impact of the destructive damage.

ES modalities also have indirect effects in multiple levels, cases and occasions, by affecting directly different populations of microbiota/microbiomes and also germ-ganisms. These are the end biological effectors in a positive or negative sense. Thus, EM modalities in destructive dosages are applicable directly against spoilage and pathogenic microorganisms. In this way, when it comes to agriculture and the food industry, they alleviate disruptive effects in many goods, especially in edible supplies. Similar applications in health promotion and restoration (human, animal, plant) include: (i) the regulatory use of microbiomes as the latter are known to sustain or restore health, and (ii) the bolstering of the efficiency of pharmabiotics as the latter are microbiome-based concoctions of therapeutic use.

Of course, there is always the causatively direct, although conceptually indirect, use of ES as antimicrobial agents proactively or reactively, *in situ, in vitro* or even *in vivo* (electrosterilization/electropasteurization/electrosanitization) in single, multiple or multi-agent regimens to counter multiple infectious diseases without the logistical tail needed for chemical/biochemical drugs.

Microbiota electrified

The extended use of antibiotics against infectious diseases, zoonoses as well as for various agricultural and environmental purposes is on the verge of abuse (English and Gaur 2010, Kleinkauf and Monnet 2013). This tendency has reinforced the natural resistance mechanisms of microbes, resulting in low efficacy and environmental burden. Similarly, synthetic preservatives have been extensively used for the preservation of perishable food products for decades, but consumers' concerns for their potentially health-compromising effects and the modern market preference for more natural and low-processed foods has fueled the search for natural antimicrobials and mild antimicrobial treatments (Skenderidis et al. 2019, Nair et al. 2020, Didaras et al. 2021).

To such concerns, it should be added that both preservatives and antibiotics seem to become harder to come by, as there is a proverbial bottleneck in the design and development of newer designs at a time when microbial variability seems to undergo explosive increase for a number of reasons like climate change, migration and transportation (that transfer and transplant massive amounts of microbiota, thus rearranging local microbiomes) and the evolutionary pressure due to the increased use of the aforementioned amenities.

Then there are several sustainability issues. The usual antimicrobial amenities come at a cost, but also with some environmental footprint: the expiration date implies a need for stocking and possibly disposing of stocks regularly; security dictates large stocks that have to be replenished when exhausted, but this actually leads to an abundance of waste when the safety margin is maintained. Recycling of stocks is not always applicable, especially against high-impact, rare-occasion agents.

The administration form, or rather the packaging, of modern pharmaceuticals produces a lot of waste and is expensive, bulky and suitable only for a specific mode of retail use—not for massive applications, when human lives are concerned. For agricultural and industrial applications, different marketing rules apply and some economies of scale are possible, but the mid-term interpretation of 'scale' tends to become 'abuse' and thus suggests a rather liberal if not ill-advised use, contradicting every concept of antibiotic chaperoning. Furthermore, antibiotics need storage and although their requirements are vastly more permissive than, say, vaccines and other biologically active compounds, such requirements are by definition unsustainable or poorly sustainable in crises, and limit the availability, readiness and distribution pipelines and efforts (Kambouris et al. 2017).

Therefore, the need for novel, better and more affordable amenities has incited research for alternative approaches. Under the guise of electromicrobiology, the use of electrostimulation (ES) modalities in different forms and shapes, occasionally termed collectively Electroceuticals (Kambouris et al. 2014) in a broader sense, promises cost-effective, adaptable and flexible solutions either as surrogates or as complements to more classical interventions (Giladi et al. 2008, Kambouris et al. 2014, 2017) but conceptually even to more groundbreaking and exotic ones, including the Traditional, Complementary and Alternative Medicinal contexts

(TCAM), which are usually more sustainable in specific spatio-temporal contexts as they use locally available resources (Kramlich 2014). Although ES applies to many and diverge classes of ailments, it is its potential in managing microbiota which is the exact scope of the field of electromicrobiology that is discussed here.

The precise role of ES in microbial growth has not yet been determined (Hristov and Perez 2011, Siamoglou et al. 2020). Electrical modalities have been tested for over a century to regulate microbial growth in order to induce specific growth routines—electroregulation—and to decontaminate objects—electrosterilisation and electropasteurization (Kermanshahi and Sailani 2005, Valle et al. 2007, Petrofsky et al. 2008). The sector has received considerable attention since 1932 (Tracy 1932), especially in the field of food science (Berovic et al. 2008, Hristov and Perez 2011), mostly for suppressive applications and enhancing the conservation of edibles and beverages (Tracy 1932, Ranalli et al. 2002). However, ES was also tested for inductive applications, primarily to achieve higher yields in microbiotic maturation of liquid and solid foodstuff, in terms of both throughput time and volume, and for more efficient growth and management of microbial cultures for such use.

The ES technology is not expensive, nor overly sophisticated; the main issue with it has always been a lack in solid and focused experimental planning with clearly defined targets and research strategy. An extensive, though not cohesive, body of research has been amassed with vastly different cultures, organisms, modalities/equipment and objectives, and it clearly substantiates the potential of such an approach (Kambouris et al. 2014, 2017, Siamoglou et al. 2020, Stathoulias et al. 2020).

Conductive amenities, where electric current is directed through the cells/organisms, result in a targeted and efficient treatment with low residual energy released to the environment, thus being associated with better sustainability and lower energy pollution. Treatment of microbial cultures with conductive amenities (see Figure 9.1) causes low electromagnetic pollution compared to the respective fields and microwaves, while allowing much more precise manipulation of the growth of different microbiota than with inductive amenities (mainly exposure to fields). The effect, especially the detrimental effect, seems to be maximized when treatment coincides with propagation phases, for dividing cells seem more susceptible to ES than growing, stable or static cells (Siamoglou et al. 2020, Stathoulias et al. 2020).

Ohmic effects, both on the target and its environment, including growth substrates (Davis et al. 1992, Kambouris et al. 2014, Siamoglou et al. 2020, Stathoulias et al. 2020), offer *a priori* advantageous conditions for suppressive purposes, thus suggesting a synergy with thermal amenities. However, it is not always so and the associations seem multi-factorial in nature. The ohmic effect may be alleviated in cold environment for example and perhaps turn advantageous for the subject organism by heightening its residual temperature near the survival optima.

Exposing cells and organisms to electrical currents for time, charge and intensity values *below* the thresholds of ohmic damage (as applicable on a case-by-case basis) can be *per se* beneficial in stimulating growth routines for the microbe (Kambouris et al. 2014, 2017, Stathoulias et al. 2020), such as multiplication/propagation at the cellular level, expansion at the colony level, primary and secondary metabolite production, and self-healing. The latter, better understood in the context of the

Electrostimulation treatment of petri dish

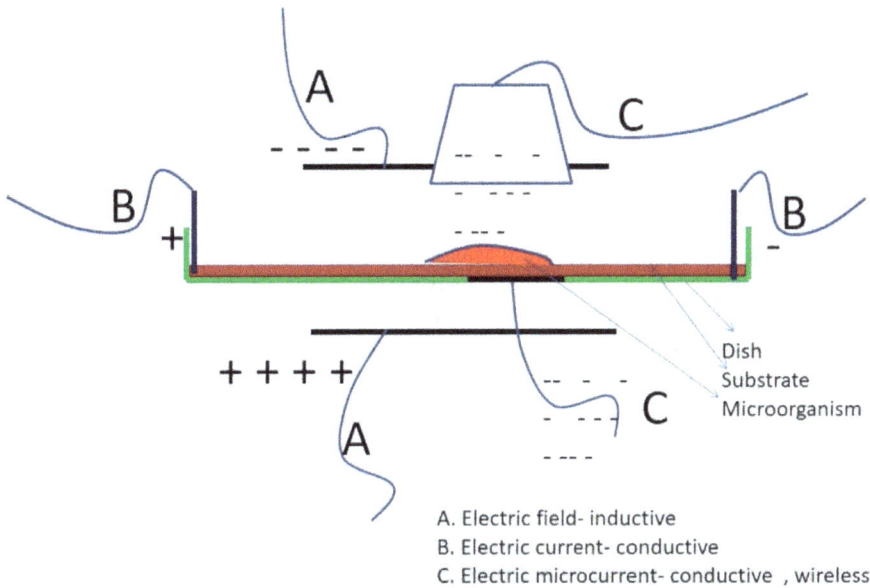

A. Electric field- inductive
B. Electric current- conductive
C. Electric microcurrent- conductive , wireless

Figure 9.1. Aggregate display of electrostimulation formats for treating a microorganism growing in a petri dish spread with nutrient substrate. (A) The inductive treatment places the object within an electric field, with various options of field being available. (B) The conductive format places electrodes in the substrate to send current through its mass; different forms of current are possible in this method. The conductive wireless method, also known as non-contact current transfer (NCCT), uses a device to ionize molecules of the air and spreads them on the treated surface, where a return electrode closes the circuit.

germ-ganism (Chapter 6), wherein microbial growth in apperceived as internally preordained and not exclusively externally dependent, is of vital importance in infection control and sterilization (Kambouris et al. 2022). This is because it is likely to undermine the effect of other amenities used in parallel or in tandem (Caubet et al. 2004). Previous experience shows that the results of ES on microbial growth may be highly diverse, depending on the microbe, and not follow linear correlations (Stathoulias et al. 2020); this observation holds water to a larger degree, especially when combining regimens. The comparative and simultaneous result of an EM amenity deliverable onto microbiota/microbiomes on or in a living host poses even more challenges, as the combined results on the two very different cellular populations could be unpredictable and antagonistic. This is the case with any stimulus enacted on a complex system, (bio)chemical drugs being a prime example, as obvious by the quest to balance efficacy and safety (Li et al. 2018). The combination of different approaches to exert control over microbial growth (not strictly antimicrobial effects), plus the combined effect of each of these amenities onto a microbe-host or microbe-environment context (not to mention a microbiome-host/environment format), is a challenge for Big Data, at least in analytical terms. Whether inclusive experimentation rather than analysis-synthesis approaches is better suited for faster results is still debatable.

Dose-response patterns are discontinuous in fungi, regarding the intensity of the DC routed through identical solid cultures of the same strain, and among different species exposed to the same treatment. Many of the observed growth differences are kinetic, rather than dynamic (Stathoulias et al. 2020). This furthers the concepts of electrodynamics and electrokinetics, compared to their original purpose, to describe the distribution, penetration and effects of electroceuticals, analogous to pharmacodynamics and pharmacokinetics (Kambouris et al. 2014, 2017).

It has been observed that when extreme conditions (such as either high or low amplitude and frequency of Alternating Current) were tested in bacterial liquid cultures and viral cell cultures, combined with mild thermal processing, a complex pattern emerged. The combination was selected because mild thermal processing is quintessential for standard biosecurity applications in the food sector, for it enhances food preservation and safety, along with savings in energy costs and carbon emissions, as opposed to high-temperature pasteurization. Additionally, it addresses problems where pathogens may be resistant to chemical treatment/deactivation due to the lack of an envelope (Kyriakopoulou et al. 2010, Iritani et al. 2014).

The antimicrobial effectiveness of the ES treatment depends mainly on its duration and the frequency, and much less on the intensity. Furthermore, external factors of importance are the combination with pasteurization (performed synchronously or asynchronously to ES) and the target microorganism. Overall, the synchronous application of pasteurization and ES offers the best microbicidal results, which, depending on the species, were up to 5 orders of magnitude higher, compared to a solely pasteurized control. Nonetheless, it should be noted that there is evidence for potentially stimulatory effects of short ES treatment schemes, which seem to enhance bacterial growth or survival during pasteurization, thus antagonizing the said established and proven antimicrobial amenities.

ES combined with heating provides better results in terms of reduction of the virus titer and inhibition of viral growth, especially at high frequency-high intensity settings of ES; however, this effect depends on the concentration of the virus as well. Under high viral titer and low frequency treatment, the opposite effect may occur, corroborating results with bacteria and fungi. Dropping, for example, the titer of viruses in environmental and food matrices (such as recreational and drinkable water, seafood, fresh produce, etc.) is of obvious applicability and could evolve into new preventive or therapeutic approaches against common viral pathogens.

On the other hand, one cannot exclude a potential stimulatory effect that low frequency ES may exert on high titers of viruses, useful in quite a few applications. Relevant examples include the enhanced production of virions to be used as vectors for vaccines, and, downstream, the increase of the efficiency of vaccines using viral vectors, to speed up the development of immunity after vaccination. The more efficient use of viral/phagal vectors for transfection in biotechnological applications and research is rather akin to the previous ones. But it must be noted that what might turn revolutionary is the possibility of increasing the efficiency of bacteriophages and virophages for the decontamination of diverse substrates (Zalewska-Piątek and Piątek 2021) or for use as biotherapeutics.

Individualizing treatment: The realm of Electroculturomics

The ability to affect the growth of microbiota, either in dynamic or in kinetic terms, may offer operational options beyond the chemical and genetic regulation of the microbiota for agro-industrial, food and pharmaceutical purposes. In all the cases, precise conditions may be necessary for achieving the expected results. Consequently, applications more amenable to precise climatic control even in massive formats (greenhouses for instance) seem more readily implementable. To establish the proper conditions and settings for the amenity, extensive and highly parallel dose-response experiments should be conducted and this is the field of Electroculturomics (Kambouris 2020, Stathoulias et al. 2020). Initially, preliminary research in the discipline would scan different EM amenities with a very limited scope of tunable parameters as offered by off-the-self equipment, methods and technology. The short-term objective would be to establish an innovative and highly promising approach to manipulate microbial growth and identify possible prospects for future development of application-specific protocols and potential directions for applied research followed by the translational, commercial dimension. A direct application of electroculturomics would be to identify potential beneficial effects for improved cultivability and enhanced growth (or survival under stress conditions) of economically important microbial cultures that produce important metabolites in fermented foods, pharmaceuticals or industrial fermentations and raw material processing or decomposition, where an optimized growth rate is of cardinal importance (Schmidt 2005, Bouki et al. 2020).

The biological activity and its underlying mechanisms are all somewhat hazy at the moment, but the diverse effects caused by the same modalities on different organisms show that a complex network of interactions should be considered at play, rather than a specific, linear pathway and a defined set of implicated genes and procedures. One may only speculate about the effects of different ES regimens per treated microbial strain/species on different growth parameters. These effects, indicatively and not exhaustively, include:

- The lag or acceleration of the onset of the exponential phase, which is of major importance in curtailing contamination and infection.

- The balancing of the increase of the biomass versus the (radial) expansion of the growth, which is critical in infection control and biomass production.

- The balance in producing primary and secondary metabolites for industrial applications (such as food and beverage industry) (Brian 1951, Perez et al. 2007, Detman et al. 2019) or catabolizing substrates in biodegradation/bioremediation applications (Kormas and Lymperopoulou 2013).

- The resistance profiles to antibiotics, antiseptics, synthetic preservatives or natural antimicrobials and other antimicrobial amenities may well recede, thus alleviating the need for new compounds. This is already observed and substantiated through the bioelectric effect (Costerton et al. 1994) that increases the microbicidal potential of antimicrobial treatments, including decontamination protocols (Davis et al. 1991) and therapeutics (Carley and Wainapel 1985, Spadaro et al. 1986, Ramadhinara and Poulas 2013, Kambouris et al. 2014).

The different windows of effects, both detrimental and beneficial, in principle allow actual targeting of specific components within a microbiome. Individualized manipulation of possible, probable or obligatory pathogens by a specific set of ES parameters might be achievable, without affecting other (beneficial) members of a microbiome, by subjecting them to intense and destructive treatment. This would be especially useful in matrices like fermented foods where pathogens or spoilage organisms need to be restricted, while starter cultures and autochthonous microbiota taking part in the fermentation process need to be unaffected or, if possible, enhanced (Bouki et al. 2020). But the principle also applies to the human microbiome in different biocompartments, especially when corrupted by aggressive, potentially pathogenic (opportunistic) strains or obligatory pathogens.

Expanding on the above, the differential susceptibility of pathogens and host tissue and organs to various ES modalities might allow wider yet selective use of electroceuticals against specific infections. Moreover, as there are many formats and a large number of electricity-based protocols already tried on different applications, including ailments (Reid and Zhao 2014), and a practically unlimited potential for developing new ones, there is an obvious issue of identifying and testing such differential applicability. Quite possibly, a range of applications wider than that for the different categories of biochemical compounds is to be expected, thus allowing multi-tasking and further increasing cost-effectiveness and sustainability, and reducing costs and environmental footprint. Still, a universal electrostimulation or electroregulation protocol is not deemed attainable, given the aforementioned issues and variability, resulting in an unrelenting need for laborious testing and development on a case-by-case basis (Stathoulias et al. 2020).

In order to resolve the mechanistic aspect of growth-related, phenotypic response to electrostimulation, the concept of electrotranscriptomics seems almost preordained, as it will elucidate initially the binary pattern in the expression of microbial genes when under electrostimulatory treatment versus untreated samples, and among different treatment protocols per sample (here, a sample must be understood as a complex entity comprising both a strain and a set of growth conditions). Consecutively, more intricate patterns, such as quantitative ones, can be dissected.

In this way, causal substantiation will bolster the empirical and descriptive observations of electroculturomics. Electrogenomics is thus likely to be the ultimate step in this phased approach, whence variations in genes and regulatory sequences will be assigned to different responses to ES stimuli, either amongst strains of the same taxon, or among different taxa. Analogous macromolecules, especially proteins, might possess different electroresponsiveness due to mutations, either directly (amino acid sequence and co-factor variance) or indirectly (conformational variance due to amino acid alterations). Actually, electrogenomics is not a brand-new concept: the basics, although not named and referred to as such, were determined earlier, when electrostimulation and electroregulation were associated with different expression rates of specific genes (Gao et al. 2005, Zhao et al. 2006, Meng et al. 2011), unfortunately without any cohesive and systematic follow-up which could firmly establish the field and further its potential.

As a discipline, electroculturomics would need some novel approaches. In order to apply EM, different culture containers are needed—from petri dishes, flasks and vials to plates, designed and manufactured to allow the effects of fields and the routing of current (Kambouris 2020, Siamoglou et al. 2020). Nanotechnology could produce highly affordable, storable and transformable products along these lines, where some of their qualities would be switched on and off according to the context of the experiment (Stathoulias et al. 2020); perhaps in a manner similar to microfluidics, in terms of the functional concept (Velegraki 2020). Such hardware would assume the functional status and shape/volume/dimensions only before use, thus allowing massive storage. Such developments are of debatable prospect, but not absolutely Sci-Fi. The cost would pose some challenges, but nothing further (Stathoulias et al. 2020).

On the other hand, integrated incubation and handling pipelines should be adapted to be compatible with instruments and setups intended for diverse EM amenities. Actually, this could be more of a challenge, especially in already operating automated solutions which would require redesign to comply with such specifications (Kambouris 2020, Siamoglou et al. 2020), as their replacement would be very costly and thus unwarranted.

The Germ-ganism under ES

The notion of the germ-ganism (Kambouris et al. 2022) refers to dispersed cell populations as parts of a single organism or, in a more dynamic context, as striving to establish a multicellular entity—the germ-ganism. This entity presents functions equivalent (similar or identical) to the ones expected from a loosely organized, distributed in space multicellular organization: regulatory arrangements, diverse development/ontogeny and self-restrained growth. The concept has been described in Chapter 6; here, it has been briefly visited in the context of Electromicrobiology.

Given that the germ-ganism, if a factuality, shows tremendous variety in form and function, it must be remembered that it occasionally consists of a multitude of very different cell subpopulations, potentially both eukaryotic and prokaryotic. The differential responsiveness of such elements to any conceivable ES stimulus must be taken for granted, as in the case of the microbiome. But the germ-ganism accounts for a higher level of integration, which must result from some sort of signal exchange. In such a case, the ES would affect the signal traffic be it by waves or by the release of chemical moieties. Usually, such interference would be *a priori* detrimental as it disrupts the exchange necessary for coordinated growth and assignment of tasks by differential regulation. As a result, some subpopulations may start growing unchecked or in a somewhat more expansive sense, and the germ-ganism may be dissolved and reassembled *de novo* with different specifications and characteristics. One prospective example is the possible degradation of quorum-sensing (QS) moieties that restrict the growth of colonies in a given set of conditions. Degrading them or altering their spatial distribution due to electrostatic attraction or repulsion would be a direct effect; changing the surface distribution of binding proteins and altering the functionality of membrane channels, in yield and position, would be an indirect way of affecting the net result of the quorum-sensing modalities. The signal would be entirely nullified/deleted or merely compromised, depending on the synergy of the abovementioned interferences and the impact on each of them per case and environment, thus forcing the germ-ganism to a different growth motif. It is understood that, depending on the new spatial pattern (or even spatio-temporal pattern) of the active signaling moieties, the growth may be actively manipulated.

Alternatively, degradation of QS signals, direct or indirect, could well result in moieties with different, perhaps opposite, functionality and thus still exerting some biological effects. Such concerns hinder the easy and prompt use of ES in therapeutics as well as in other applications, as the considerations are too many and border on Big Data. To this, one should add the consideration of the EM modalities as a factor to positively or negatively regulate, in essence to promote or forestall Programmed Cell Death (PCD) in both prokaryotic and eukaryotic microorganisms, processes that are essential for shaping different forms of the latter, some of them clearly reminiscent of the quintessence of a germ-ganism (like biofilms) and others less so (bacterial sporulation), but always implying some sort of biological logic—collective, centralized or dispersed (Hammer 2018).

The possibility to dissolve a germ-ganism to smaller ones or to a mass of independent cells would be nothing short of revolutionary in applied biology and may account for some cases of biofilm dissolution by such modalities (Kambouris et al. 2017, Patrinos et al. 2020, Siamoglou et al. 2020). It is possible that the biochemical signaling would be compromised and hence sessile forms would transform into planktonic forms, thus detaching from surfaces and becoming more susceptible to diluted/dispersed biochemical agents, these being toxic or, less frequently, beneficial. The dissolution of biofilms disinfects the tooling and infrastructure, thus safeguarding public health and the volume and quality of production in many sectors. On the other hand, creating biofilms may have a range of applications: a biofilm may be a flexible barrier to shut off toxins from tissues, degenerative enzymes and metabolites such as pH modifiers from artefacts and also from degradable products or produce. In embiomechanics, biofilms could be used as isolation/insulation matterial in micro- and nanomaterials. Furthermore, in applications such as biorestoration, biofilms may form a barrier to isolate contaminated surfaces, while the microorganisms degrade the toxins and decontaminate them. The prospect of similar effects on tumors would be just as intriguing; the core function would be their physical dissolution or at least mechanical loosening so as to expose deeply seated cells, including the meddlesome persister cells, to simultaneous access and neutralization by cytotoxic autologous and xenologous modalities.

The advanced cybernetic approach to combine the effects of a positive and a negative signal of dissimilar nature, and thus non-interfering with each other, implies a higher degree of authority and precision in the control process. Affecting the rearrangement of the microbiota that make up a germ-ganism would allow a leverage in manipulating microbial populations far more effective than any similar effect exercised directly onto the individual cells. This implies that a range of more demanding interventions comes within reach. The diverse combinations of the available signals (sorted by nature only and not by their exact form) through the bioelectric effect allow a massive range of settings: the biochemical moieties may exercise direct effect on the cell or indirect effect on the signals; the EM may do exactly the same, resulting in four basic combinations of the two categories. These combinations may promote synergy or avoid antagonism in effects on the subjects, or be used for more precise enterprises, similar to multichannel EM command systems. This could be used to suppress hostile populations, microbiomes and germ-ganisms (pathogenic, spoilage, degrading) or to boost beneficial ones (symbiotic, protective, productive). Moreover, it would allow morphing colonization and growth to suit spatio-temporal realities and specifications, and thus increase the applicability of biopharmaceuticals in medicinal, industrial and environmental setups. But the most intriguing possibility is the differential manipulation of different populations of the same microbiome/germ-ganism, which may shape the living environment to specs, and thus alleviate the unintended or reverse effects of administering a given moiety (of whatever nature) to a spatially defined but multispecies microbiome.

Increasing the yield of honest toil

The disruption of supply chains, especially due to anti-propagation measures implemented in pandemics, highlights the need for a degree of self-sufficiency within geographical units (Lugo-Morin 2020, Sarkar et al. 2021). There is some obvious escalation of the breakdown of transportation, while the breakdown of communications (or their degradation) is a direct or indirect effect at some later level of the said escalation. The impact of an epidemic may be the deletion of whole grids on the map, especially in the case of agricultural concerns, which are rated lower in healthcare priority despite the One Health concept (Magouras et al. 2020). Agricultural units may be extremely extensive in spatial terms and intensively exploited to achieve market sufficiency at a profit (van Bruggen et al. 2019). Intense exploitations use genetically identical plants, clones of the same cultivar (Wieczorek and Wright 2012). This homogeneity in a given large and dense population allows prompt dissemination of a pathogen within the said population over long distances (Yoshida et al. 2013, Goss et al. 2014). Given that Diversity is an asset in prospectively safeguarding from Chance events (Kourilsky 2016), the emergence of better adapted pathogens may be considered as one example of such chance events.

The deletion, at least functional, of a grid on the map is truly an extreme scenario but not an improbable one. The isolation to curtail the dispersion of a highly contagious agent is, after the COVID-19 pandemic, a Standard Operating Procedure (SOP) exemplified by quarantine or lockdown and actually implemented with less reservation than expected in both cases. It can always be substantiated as an improvement in prospect, difficult to prove but impossible to dismiss, compared with non-implementation of such measures. It is also very lucrative for many concerns, and speculation on the subject would be factored in for many different activities, insurances included.

When it comes to agricultural production in an isolated or semi-isolated region due to traffic limitations (the term "traffic" should be understood to include, without being restricted to, trade, transportation and travel), such disruptions may cause physically and financially significant if not catastrophic detrimental effects. In plant exploitation, this is due to the high volume of chemical fertilizers and biocides required for optimizing the yield, the former especially for enhancing the rather poor and/or intensively cultivated small plots, possibly in labor-intensive formats, but also in highly automated ones. The use of such fertilizers could be supplemented or, ideally, substituted by other, cleaner approaches, requiring less off-area transportation and ideally without a disproportionate environmental footprint, while offering a positive cost-effectiveness ratio in both normal and emergency conditions. If such amenities were to be materialized, a more robust and resilient production process could be expected, capable of sustaining the local communities and, to a second degree, upkeeping an income through commerce, should the marketing networks remain operative to a degree. Electromagnetic amenities have been tried repeatedly, with excellent results, in this respect, mainly by treating seeds (De Souza et al. 2006, Efthimiadou et al. 2014, Katsenios et al. 2016) and by using magnetized water for irrigation (Hilal et al. 2002, Maheshwari and Singh Grewal 2009, Sarraf et al. 2020). If the approach is based on *in-situ*, such as solar, energy production and combined with local varieties adapted to low-fertility soil and low demands in irrigation/water consumption, a better yield might be achievable with minimal chemical and energy input and some organic recycling.

The latter is vital in a limited-waste agricultural economy, which is not directly associated with biosecurity but makes the application of biosecurity more affordable and easier to enact as it increases sustainability (see Chapter 2). In this concept, the increased volume of the green parts of the plants, the ones not suitable for human consumption, can be used as fodder for flocks of productive animals of local varieties that produce high-quality milk and are well-adapted to free pastures for millennia in these localities and climates (Staglianò et al. 2005), and which may also produce manure to close the circle. The produced goods qualify for biological agriculture as electromagnetism and magnetically enhanced water irrigation are not considered non-biological-agriculture-compatible amenities and means; thus, higher prices can be sought in normal conditions, while the low content of water allows keeping the crops unrefrigerated and still unmolested for longer periods, at least locally and in limited quantities such as a household's provisions, thus resulting in no loss of food or depreciation due to lower market access rates.

To this scheme, the different classes of biocides can be also replaced by a robust EM approach. Such chemical amenities, and occasionally biologicals/biochemicals, are costly and voluminous, require transportation resources for access and delivery, and produce massive negative environmental footprint. A combined regimen that would fulfil both the tasks of production enhancement and disease control would be the Holy Grail in agriculture—a boost to inherent biosecurity and bioresilience compliance. It would also reduce the expenditure per production unit in monetary and resource terms, and improve the sustainability and environmental-friendliness of the exploitation. Should the improvements in pest control and yield make genetic modification superfluous or obviate it, and instead promote local varieties, species and cultivars, the long-term sustainability and bioresilience/biosecurity would increase even further, by eliminating the factor of genetic pollution. The better adaptation of local varieties means less need for tending and higher accumulated experience and expertise, thus minimising risks and improving the overall cost-effectiveness.

Furthermore, the management of the soil microbiome could assist in both cases, yield and protection of plant and animal capital, given that the microbiome may increase the fertility of the soil or the growth/metabolism of an animal and keep a number of prospective pathogens in check by antagonising them or by creating the biochemical environment which keeps them in relative harmony with the host. It needs to be further tested whether the above interactions may also reduce the relative water consumption.

The pre-plantation enhancement of seeds has been previously tried with magnetic exposure by using a compact device (Efthimiadou et al. 2014, Katsenios et al. 2016). It is still too heavy and expensive to be used in individual or even strictly local conditions, but suitable for larger, massive exploitations or in administratively centralized formats, for treating higher volumes of seeds and perhaps water (Abou El-Yazied et al. 2012) and conceivably combining medical and agricultural use (Katsenios et al. 2016). Such a device may be procured collectively by a number of small local farmers to successively treat their reproductive material and possibly quantities of water used for the irrigation of these species. In this way, higher yields can be achieved with small upfront and minimal recurring costs, as the basic amenity would be electricity, available in an urban context where the seed may be treated without the need for deploying any device and thus power generation in or near the fields.

Still, what is needed is portable devices, preferably similar in physical dimensions to the ones previously described in the context of culturomics (Stathoulias et al. 2020), that allow flexible applications in warmhouses and open field conditions. Settings among treatment regimens for different species may vary, but the principle of the underlying biological mechanism should be generic and, thus, the issue of adapting to a given exploitation would be a matter of fine-tuning and optimization. In the same context, a generalized application of only electric, not magnetic, treatment may be preferable; this would allow more precise attuning of the bioactive amenity, as treatment by magnetic fields is much more susceptible to interference and a small diversion from the standardized procedure may result in drastic changes in output (Siamoglou et al. 2020). Also, suboptimal handling is to be expected at the hands of producers who have no technical infrastructure or scientific and experimental training.

Another operational approach would be to develop and field multivalent, multiple-output instruments. Such devices would ideally offer different settings for producing magnetic and electric fields and delivering currents. The latter seems distant and rather costly to implement massively outdoors; yet, massive fielding would curtail design, development and production costs for bulk purchases, while the capability for different amenities in a single instrument would provide alternatives if a procedure or protocol is proven unsuitable, making a drastically different set of options available, thus increasing the resilience of the method in unexpected and evolutionary contexts. Such instruments may be purchased centrally and in bulk, for better prices, and then distributed to different geographical locations where the end users would own them collectively and circulate them amongst the ones who would have subsidized the purchase in an area.

Irrespective of the device and its size, cost and principle, the great enabler in strictly local settings is the familiarization of interested parties/producers with commercial IT technologies through everyday use. This will be helpful in their long-distance, synchronous or asynchronous training and support, necessary for properly executing the different steps of the treatment procedures and troubleshooting. The new generation of farmers (meant in cultural and not biological terms) is well-acquainted with Internet-based amenities and became more so during the pandemic. Thus, a networking community for sharing and support would further and accelerate the beneficial impact.

References

Abou El-Yazied, A. et al. (2012). Effect of magnetic field treatments for seeds and irrigation water as well as N, P and K levels on productivity of tomato plants. Journal of Applied Sciences Research, 8(4): 2088–2099.

Berovic, M. et al. (2008). The influence of galvanic field on Saccharomyces cerevisiae in grape must fermentation. Vitis, 47(2): 117–122. doi: 10.5073/VITIS.2008.47.117-122.

Bouki, P. et al. (2020). Microbiomic prospects in fermented food and beverage technology. pp. 245–277. *In*: Kambouris, M.E. and Velegraki, A. (eds.). Microbiomics: Dimensions, Applications, and Translational Implications of Human and Environmental Microbiome Research. Elsevier. doi: 10.1016/B978-0-12-816664-2.00012-8.

Brian, P.W. (1951). Antibiotics produced by fungi. The Botanical Review, 17(6): 357–430. doi: 10.1007/BF02879038.

van Bruggen, A.H.C. et al. (2019). One Health - Cycling of diverse microbial communities as a connecting force for soil, plant, animal, human and ecosystem health. Science of the Total Environment. Elsevier B.V., pp. 927–937. doi: 10.1016/j.scitotenv.2019.02.091.

Carley, P.J. and Wainapel, S.F. (1985). Electrotherapy for acceleration of wound healing: Low intensity direct current. Archives of physical medicine and rehabilitation, 66(7): 443–446.

Caubet, R. et al. (2004). A radio frequency electric current enhances antibiotic efficacy against bacterial biofilms. Antimicrobial Agents and Chemotherapy, 48(12): 4662–4664. doi: 10.1128/AAC.48.12.4662-4664.2004.

Costerton, J.W. et al. (1994). Mechanism of electrical enhancement of efficacy of antibiotics in killing biofilm bacteria. Antimicrobial Agents and Chemotherapy, 38(12): 2803–2809. doi: 10.1128/AAC.38.12.2803.

Davis, C.P. et al. (1991). Bacterial and fungal killing by iontophoresis with long-lived electrodes. Antimicrobial Agents and Chemotherapy, 35(10): 2131–2134. doi: 10.1128/AAC.35.10.2131.

Davis, C.P. et al. (1992). Iontophoresis generates an antimicrobial effect that remains after iontophoresis ceases. Antimicrobial Agents and Chemotherapy, 36(11): 2552–2555. doi: 10.1128/AAC.36.11.2552.

Detman, A. et al. (2019). Cell factories converting lactate and acetate to butyrate: *Clostridium butyricum* and microbial communities from dark fermentation bioreactors. Microbial Cell Factories, 18(1): 36. doi: 10.1186/s12934-019-1085-1.

Didaras, N.A. et al. (2021). Biological properties of bee bread collected from apiaries located across Greece. Antibiotics, 10(5). doi: 10.3390/ANTIBIOTICS10050555.

Efthimiadou, A. et al. (2014). Effects of presowing pulsed electromagnetic treatment of tomato seed on growth, yield, and lycopene content. Scientific World Journal, 2014: 369745. doi: 10.1155/2014/369745.

English, B.K. and Gaur, A.H. (2010). The use and abuse of antibiotics and the development of antibiotic resistance. Advances in Experimental Medicine and Biology, 659: 73–82. doi: 10.1007/978-1-4419-0981-7_6.

Gao, W. et al. (2005). Effects of a strong static magnetic field on bacterium Shewanella oneidensis: An assessment by using whole genome microarray. Bioelectromagnetics, 26(7): 558–563. doi: 10.1002/bem.20133.

Giladi, M. et al. (2008). Microbial growth inhibition by alternating electric fields. Antimicrobial Agents and Chemotherapy, 52(10): 3517–3522. doi: 10.1128/AAC.00673-08.

Goss, E.M. et al. (2014). The Irish potato famine pathogen Phytophthora infestans originated in central Mexico rather than the Andes. Proceedings of the National Academy of Sciences, 111(24): 8791–8796. doi: 10.1073/pnas.1401884111.

Hammer, N.D. (2018). Microbial programmed cell death. Apoptosis and Beyond: The Many Ways Cells Die. John Wiley & Sons, Ltd, pp. 49–70. doi: 10.1002/9781119432463.CH3.

Hilal, M.H. et al. (2002). Application of magnetic technologies in desert agriculture: III. Effect of magnetized water on yield and uptake of certain elements by citrus in relation to nutrients mobilization in soil. Egyptian Journal of Soil Science, 42(1): 43–56.

Hristov, J. and Perez, V. (2011). Critical analysis of data concerning Saccharomyces cerevisiae free-cell proliferations and fermentations assisted by magnetic and electromagnetic fields. International Review of Chemical Engineering, 3(1): 3–20.

Iritani, N. et al. (2014). Detection and genetic characterization of human enteric viruses in oyster-associated gastroenteritis outbreaks between 2001 and 2012 in Osaka City, Japan. Journal of Medical Virology, 86(12): 2019–2025. doi: 10.1002/JMV.23883.

Kambouris, M. et al. (2014). From therapeutic Electrotherapy to Electroceuticals: Formats, Applications and Prospects of Electrostimulation. Annual Research & Review in Biology, 4(20): 3054–3070. doi: 10.9734/arrb/2014/10563.

Kambouris, M.E. et al. (2017). Wireless electrostimulation: A new approach in combating infection? Future Microbiology, 12(3): 255–65. doi: 10.2217/fmb-2017-0157.

Kambouris, M.E. (2020). Culturomics: The Alternative From the Past. pp. 155–173. *In*: Kambouris, M.E. and Velegraki, A. (eds.). Microbiomics: Dimensions, Applications, and Translational Implications of Human and Environmental Microbiome Research. Elsevier, doi: 10.1016/b978-0-12-816664-2.00008-6.

Kambouris, M.E. et al. (2022). Beyond the microbiome: Germ-ganism? An Integrative Idea for Microbial Existence, Organization, Growth, Pathogenicity, and Therapeutics', Omics : A Journal of Integrative Biology, 26(4): 204–217. doi: 10.1089/OMI.2022.0015.

Katsenios, N. et al. (2016). Role of pulsed electromagnetic field on enzyme activity, germination, plant growth and yield of durum wheat. Biocatalysis and Agricultural Biotechnology, 6: 152–158. doi: 10.1016/J.BCAB.2016.03.010.

Kermanshahi, R.K. and Sailani, M.R. (2005). Effect of static electric field treatment on multiple antibiotic-resistant pathogenic strains of *Escherichia coli* and *Staphylococcus aureus*. Journal of Microbiology, Immunology, and Infection, 38(6): 394–398.

Kleinkauf, N. et al. (2013). Risk assessment on the impact of environmental usage of triazoles on the development and spread of resistance to medical triazoles in *Aspergillus* species. Stockholm ECDC.

Kormas, K.A. and Lymperopoulou, D.S. (2013). Cyanobacterial toxin degrading bacteria: Who are they? BioMed Research International, 2013: 463894. doi: 10.1155/2013/463894.

Kourilsky, P. (2016). The natural defense system and the normative self model. F1000Research, 5: 797. doi: 10.12688/F1000RESEARCH.8518.1.

Kramlich, D. (2014). Introduction to complementary, alternative, and traditional therapies. Critical Care Nurse, 34(6): 50–6; quiz 57. doi: 10.4037/ccn2014807.

Kyriakopoulou, Z. et al. (2010). Molecular identification and full genome analysis of an echovirus 7 strain isolated from the environment in Greece. Virus Genes, 40(2): 183–192. doi: 10.1007/S11262-009-0446 Y.

Li, X.X. et al. (2018). Determining the balance between drug efficacy and safety by the network and biological system profile of its therapeutic target. Frontiers in Pharmacology, 9: 1245. doi: 10.3389/FPHAR.2018.01245/BIBTEX.

Lugo-Morin, D.R. (2020). Global Food Security in a Pandemic: The Case of the New Coronavirus (COVID-19)', World, 1(2): 171–190. doi: 10.3390/WORLD1020013.

Magouras, I. et al. (2020). Emerging zoonotic diseases: Should we rethink the animal–human interface? Frontiers in Veterinary Science, 7: 582743. doi: 10.3389/FVETS.2020.582743/BIBTEX.

Maheshwari, B.L. and Singh Grewal, H. (2009). Magnetic treatment of irrigation water: Its effects on vegetable crop yield and water productivity. Agricultural Water Management, 96(8): 1229–1236. doi: 10.1016/j.agwat.2009.03.016.

Meng, S. et al. (2011). Chapter 3. Electrical stimulation in tissue regeneration. *In*: Gargiulo, G.D. and McEwan, A. (eds.). Applied Biomedical Engineering. InTech. doi: 10.5772/18874.

Nair, A. et al. (2020). Harnessing the antibacterial activity of Quercus infectoria and Phyllanthus emblica against antibiotic-resistant Salmonella Typhi and Salmonella Enteritidis of poultry origin. Veterinary World, 13(7): 1388. doi: 10.14202/VETWORLD.2020.1388-1396.

Patrinos, G.P. et al. (2020). Bacteriome and Archaeome: The core family under the microbiomic roof. In Kambouris, M. and Velegraki, A. (eds.). Microbiomics: Dimensions, Applications, and Translational Implications of Human and Environmental Microbiome Research. ELSEVIER ACADEMIC PRESS.

Perez, V.H. et al. (2007). Bioreactor coupled with electromagnetic field generator: Effects of extremely low frequency electromagnetic fields on ethanol production by *Saccharomyces cerevisiae*. Biotechnology Progress, 23(5): 1091–1094. doi: 10.1021/bp070078k.

Petrofsky, J. et al. (2008). Effect of electrical stimulation on bacterial growth. J Neurolog Orthop Med Surg, 31: 43–49.

Ramadhinara, A. and Poulas, K. (2013). Use of wireless microcurrent stimulation for the treatment of diabetes-related wounds: 2 case reports. Advances in Skin and Wound Care, 26(1): 1–4. doi: 10.1097/01.ASW.0000425942.32993.e9.

Ranalli, G. et al. (2002). Effects of low electric treatment on yeast microflora. Journal of Applied Microbiology, 93(5): 877–883. doi: 10.1046/j.1365-2672.2002.01758.x.

Reid, B. and Zhao, M. (2014). The electrical response to injury: Molecular mechanisms and wound healing. Advances in Wound Care, 3(2): 184. doi: 10.1089/WOUND.2013.0442.

Sarkar, A. et al. (2021). Evaluation of the determinants of food security within the COVID-19 pandemic circumstances—a particular case of Shaanxi, China. Global Health Research and Policy, 6(1): 1–11. doi: 10.1186/S41256-021-00230-2/FIGURES/2.

Sarraf, M. et al. (2020). Magnetic Field (MF) Applications in plants: An overview. Plants, 9(9): 1139. doi: 10.3390/PLANTS9091139.

Schmidt, F. (2005). Optimization and scale up of industrial fermentation processes. Applied Microbiology and Biotechnology, 68(4): 425–435. doi: 10.1007/S00253-005-0003-0.

Siamoglou, S. et al. (2020). Electromagnetism and the microbiome(s). pp. 299–331. *In*: Kambouris, M.E. and Velegraki, A. (eds.). Microbiomics: Dimensions, Applications, and Translational Implications of Human and Environmental Microbiome Research. ELSEVIER ACADEMIC PRESS.

Skenderidis, P. et al. (2019). The *in vitro* antimicrobial activity assessment of ultrasound assisted Lycium barbarum fruit extracts and pomegranate fruit peels. Journal of Food Measurement and Characterization, 13(3): 2017–2031. doi: 10.1007/S11694-019-00123-6.

De Souza, A. et al. (2006). Pre-sowing magnetic treatments of tomato seeds increase the growth and yield of plants. Bioelectromagnetics, 27(4): 247–257. doi: 10.1002/BEM.20206.

Spadaro, J.A. et al. (1986). Bacterial inhibition by electrical activation of percutaneous silver implants. Journal of Biomedical Materials Research, 20(5): 565–577. doi: 10.1002/jbm.820200504.

Staglianò, N. et al. (2005). Mediterranean pastures management by local cattle breeds for the valorization of typical products and for the development of nature tourism. *In*: Molina, A. et al. (eds.). Sustainable Grazing, Nutritional Utilization and Quality of Sheep and Goat Products. (Options Méditerranéennes : Série A. Séminaires Méditerranéens; n. 67. Zaragoza: CIHEAM, pp. 239–244.

Stathoulias, A. et al. (2020). Toward high-throughput fungal electroculturomics and new Omics methodologies in 21st-Century Microbiology and Ecology. OMICS A Journal of Integrative Biology, 24(8): 493–504. doi: 10.1089/omi.2020.0012.

Tracy, R.L. (1932). Lethal effect of alternating current on yeast cells 1. Journal of Bacteriology, 24(6): 423–438. doi: 10.1128/jb.24.6.423-438.1932.

Valle, A. et al. (2007). Effects of low electric current (LEC) treatment on pure bacterial cultures. Journal of Applied Microbiology, 103(5): 1376–1385. doi: 10.1111/j.1365-2672.2007.03374.x.

Velegraki, A. (2020). Panmicrobial Microarrays. *In*: Kambouris, M.E. and Velegraki, A. (eds.). Microbiomics: Dimensions, Applications, and Translational Implications of Human and Environmental Microbiome Research. ELSEVIER ACADEMIC PRESS, pp. 95–120.

Wieczorek, A.M. and Wright, M.G. (2012). History of agricultural biotechnology: How crop development has evolved. Nature Education Knowledge, 3(10): 9.

Yoshida, K. et al. (2013). The rise and fall of the Phytophthora infestans lineage that triggered the Irish potato famine. eLife, 2013(2): e00731. doi: 10.7554/eLife.00731.

Zalewska-Piątek, B. and Piątek, R. (2021). Bacteriophages as potential tools for use in antimicrobial therapy and vaccine development. Pharmaceuticals, 14(4): 331. doi: 10.3390/PH14040331.

Zhao, M. et al. (2006). Electrical signals control wound healing through phosphatidylinositol-3-OH kinase-γ and PTEN. Nature, 442(7101): 457–460. doi: 10.1038/nature04925.

10

Wars, Crime and Terror
The Perpetrated Dimension of Biothreats

George D. Kostis[1] and *Manousos E. Kambouris*[2,*]

Introduction

War is a stern and violent teacher and humanity still has a lot to learn. To discuss theories concerning crime, terrorism and war, it is a prerequisite to have the above notions clarified so as to have them critically applied in the 'bio' context. Basically, they are used haphazardly by the arbitrary global audience, since war can be tantamount to terrorism for someone and crime for someone else. Many efforts to approach these relevant matters have not solved the riddles of the specific notions, and the collective effort does not seem to alleviate tensions, but rather prompt the world to extinction at an increasingly dangerous pace.

Times do change, and the rules with them. No matter how much anyone want to believe that war has been reduced to the blood-stained pages of history books, preferably slung to oblivion and shortly belonging to a forgotten past, the reality is anything but that. The recent conflict in Eastern Europe and its repercussions (like the ever-increasing tensions in the World) show beyond the shadow of a doubt that war is still here, playing a decisive role in the political, social, economic and strategic affairs of the world.

Within this context, we must understand that war is not of a static and stable disposition but rather of a dynamic one. Terrorism, a phenomenon blossoming since the mid-20th century but in actuality subtly present throughout history, is not just

[1] Hellenic Army Academy, Vari Greece.
   Email: george.d.kostis@gmail.com
[2] University of Patras, School of Health Sciences, Department of Pharmacy, Patras, Greece & The Golden Helix Foundation, London, United Kingdom.
* Corresponding author: mekambouris@yahoo.com

another (level of) crime meant to be tackled by the Common Criminal Law enhanced with additional respective provisions and means, but rather leans onto another form of war, occasionally almost a declared one.

The most formidable enemies that modern states have to face for the majority of the official states of the UN, at least until 2022, were not other countries or rather states, like in the past. They were, occasionally are and very probably will be, Non-State Actors, including but not limited to designated terrorist groups, possibly partially conscripting from the underworld—national or international societies of crime. Other such non-state players may be international or multinational mega-corporations.

Nothing mentioned above is strictly novel. The *Hassassin* (Britannica n.d. a) were an accomplished terror group in the Muslim world that spread to Europe after the Crusades; the Templars (Britannica n.d. b) were conceived as exactly such a threat by France, irrespective of any ulterior motives. Companies like the Dutch West India Company and the British East India Company (Britannica n.d. c, d) come to mind as cases of private interests fostering wars against states/nations, notionally, or rather almost, without direct state involvement in the aggression. More recently, relevant examples include mining concerns or trusts involved in the disgrace of the Banana Republics (Wikipedia n.d.), which made a joke of the prerogatives of the UN and the League of Nations before it.

Such fluid and elusive entities are capable of inflicting decisive blows by striking against vulnerable targets at key points. This undermines a citizen's trust on the state and thus irreparably shakes the foundations of modern societies, both developed and developing.

The current chapter cannot be approached exclusively in terms of theory, tracking answers and following the causality of things. It cannot depend on any notion of strategy reduced to the simple but perfectly inclusive 'ends, ways and means' prerogative, which indeed governs every military—and not only military—venture. It will draw on the practical and realistic dimensions of the matter and will ideally answer the fundamental questions.

War, crime and terrorism: the Biological dimension

Fundamentally, war is described as 'a situation in which there is aggressive competition between groups, companies, countries over a period of time'; the definition of armed conflicts, as given by the International Court of Justice after the war in the former Yugoslavia during the Tadiç Appeal, is presented in Box 10.1.

Crime, on the other hand, is defined as 'acts or omissions forbidden by law' (Sowmyya 2011). War is a situation and is enacted after a declaration of war has been issued by one state (or side) to another, a tradition that is rarely followed nowadays.

Unfortunately, the lack of a clear definition of terms such as 'terrorism' is usually exploited not only by governments but also by the terrorists themselves. The fact that *"one man's terrorist is another man's freedom fighter"* (Ganor 2010) is a paradox that causes even more confusion among academic circles in the international anarchical society (Box 10.2). Since the affairs of states are by definition not subject to any juridical authority and are thus anarchical in the sense of the lack of any

---

Box 10.1

(1) An armed conflict exists whenever there is a resort to armed force between States or protracted armed violence between governmental authorities and organized armed groups or between such groups within a State. These hostilities [like in the former Yugoslavia] exceed the criteria of intensity required in both international and non-international armed conflicts. There has been prolonged, large-scale violence between the armed forces of various States and between government forces and organized rebel groups.

(2) War in terms of legislation has the exact same meaning both at national and international levels. Crime at an international level has to do with serious offenses that violate the Law of Armed Conflict (war crimes), the International Humanitarian Law (crimes against humanity and genocides) and the commiting of violence (Crime of Aggression).

(3) Aggression is recognized as a crime according to Article 8 of Charter of the Statute of the International Court of Justice:

ARTICLE 8: Crime of aggression

1. For the purpose of this Statute, "crime of aggression" means the planning, preparation, initiation or execution, by a person in a position effectively to exercise control over or to direct the political or military action of a State, of an act of aggression which, by its character, gravity and scale, constitutes a manifest violation of the Charter of the United Nations.

ARTICLE 8bis: War crimes

Among others "For the purpose of this Statute, 'war crimes' means:

Employing poison or poisoned weapons;

Employing asphyxiating, poisonous or other gases, and all analogous liquids, materials or devices;

Employing bullets which expand or flatten easily in the human body, such as bullets with a hard envelope which does not entirely cover the core or is pierced with incisions;

Employing weapons, projectiles and material and methods of warfare which are of a nature to cause superfluous injury or unnecessary suffering or which are inherently indiscriminate in violation of the international law of armed conflict, provided that such weapons, projectiles and material and methods of warfare are the subject of a comprehensive prohibition and are included in an annex to this Statute, by an amendment in accordance with the relevant provisions set forth in articles 121 and 123.

---

subjugation by some supreme authority (benign anarchy), it is a playground of perpetual violence, bullying and lawlessness always ready to drift to malign anarchy understood as chaos (Lechner 2017).

Box 10.2

According to the UN Security Council Resolution 1566 of 2004, the United Nations define Terrorism as "criminal acts, including against civilians, committed with the intent to cause death or serious bodily injury, or taking of hostages, with the purpose to provoke a state of terror in the general public or in a group of persons or particular persons, intimidate a population or compel a government or an international organization to do or to abstain from doing any act".

The definition given by the U.S. Army Manual states that terrorism is the "calculated use of unlawful violence or threat of unlawful violence to inculcate fear. It is intended to coerce or intimidate governments or societies to attain political, religious, or ideological goals."

The real problem arises from the complex relation of terrorism to war and crime. The confusion between armed conflicts and terrorism is a very commonplace phenomenon, given the fact that wars are often described as terrorist acts and the militants/combatants participating in these acts are often treated as terrorists, especially in case of non-declaration-of-war armed conflicts, which has been the norm for at least 60 years now. This situation makes the effective application of the active legislation even harder and, as a result, the fight against terrorism is not as effective as it would have been in a different situation.

Nevertheless, there are some distinct boundaries with which terrorism can be differentiated from an official or even normal version of armed conflict; in case of the latter, the law of armed conflict, and the doctrines of Geneva and Hague Agreements are applied, according to which acts of violence are not considered to be terrorist or criminal acts. On the contrary, among the main characteristics of terrorist acts is the fact that terrorist attacks happen in peacetime and are prosecuted according to either the national or the international criminal laws (Belandis 2004).

Similarly, the boundaries between terrorism and common crime are even more discernible; when it comes to crime, violence is committed by the subject to achieve a certain profit—material or non-material—for oneself, while the object of this offensive is the victim by definition, without the verdict of a conflict hanging in the balance. The main indirect objective of terrorism though is to pass a message to the public through a violent act in order to weaken or even overthrow the current social *status quo* (Hoffman 2017). This act of violence has a two-fold goal: first a direct, physical effect, namely the potential to inflict mass casualties and/or cause disruption. The second goal is the indirect effect, by causing psychological injuries which may equal or even surpass the direct effects in terms of impact.

The confusion and overlap of these terms are exacerbated by the element of biological causality or agency. For example, engaging in biological warfare, usually understood as "the use of biological agents during periods of war to cause disease among enemy soldiers or among crops in enemy countries" (Box 10.1), is a war crime.

The perpetrated events of biological causality, casually and collectively referred to as a 'bioattack', are currently classified, as mentioned previously, under three major labels: biocrime, bioterrorism and biowarfare (occasionally dubbed as '3B'). The classification is effected by the nature of the perpetrator and the intended impact. They may be classified by the agent and, conditionally, by the target. Targeting any part of the agricultural sector, from fishery to orchards and from wild game to intensive farming (breeding/culturing), is the realm of agroterrorism (see Chapter 2). The events of this kind are almost always massive (a) because only through massive impact can they have any appreciable detrimental (factual or prospective) effect, (b) due to the far less resilience afforded by surveillance and regulatory authorities to non-human populations, if for no other reason, due to the lack of vocal communication between prospective patients and the overseer of health promotion, and (c) since the conditions, especially in agricultural exploitations and even more so in intensive ones, actively promote transmission, as mentioned in previous chapters (i.e., see Chapters 2 and 9).

The legal demarcation between terrorism and crime usually lies with the fact that the former has a high impact and ideological dimension, whereas the latter has a relatively low impact and profit-driven motivation (profit taken *sensu lato* and including revenge). There are many issues with these definitions, as terrorism is a capital crime in many legal systems and this also extends to warfare and armed conflict .However, in the end, a biocrime is not expected to escalate to a Global Catastrophic BioRisk (GCBR) level, while bioterrorism is, sometimes even unintentionally (Kambouris et al. 2018, Kambouris 2021a, c).

Exploring the agents

The definitions of a perpetrated biothreat (that is, bioattack) based on microbiological entities (biocrime-bioterrorism-biowarfare) are somewhat restrictive. Conceptually, biowarfare as well as bioterrorism and biocrime are not limited in scope to the microbiome. The microbiological warfare, or germ warfare, is simply the most common means. Biochemical warfare, where biomolecules are used in cell-free formats like biotoxins and bioregulators (to a far lesser degree), is also known in depth and well understood, being a part of biowarfare, with a number of attributes of chemical warfare—in terms of robustness of agents, detection/classification and decontamination approaches and non-replicative, non-propagating nature of the said agents, where carryover transmission depletes the local active concentration and leads to functional decay of the agent, similarly to radiological events.

Germ warfare and biochemical warfare are not the only forms of biowarfare. Before continuing, one must underscore the fact that toxin warfare is occasionally used as a surrogate term for biochemical warfare, to underline the causative nature of biotoxins in many, if not most, cases; in actuality, this is slightly erroneous, for toxins do exist beyond the realm of biotoxins: chemical toxins, especially inorganic toxins such as Arsenic and radiotoxins (Thallium being a well-known example), must be included (Boltsis et al. 2021). The term 'toxin' indicates that the target/object is biological, while the effector may be biological (biotoxin), radiological (radiotoxin) or chemical (chemotoxin or simply toxin). The term toxin alone may refer to any of the three, especially in an agnostic or inclusive context. There are other biological, chemical and radiological agents used in terrorist, criminal and warfare applications as well, that do not have toxic effects; such are substances with corrosive effects (Kip and Van Veen 2015), and this is only one example. The attack against technidal items (Kambouris and Georgoulas 2021, Kambouris 2021b) by biological agents, long known to degrade artefacts, textiles, provisions and structural materials (especially timber), is already identified as an option (Gottschalk and Preiser 2005). It carries significant potential for future use through optimized microbial strains, especially custom-engineered xenobiota (as mentioned in Chapter 4), or innovative remakes— of purely intentional character—of the well-known biblical incident of an army rendered weaponless due to rodents degrading the leather straps of arms and armor (Dawson 1925). In such a capacity, one could consider the advent of anti-material bioagents (Gottschalk and Preiser 2005) and speculate that modified versions of strains used for biomining could be dispersed or sprayed to corrode and thus degrade the performance of important parts of hardware. For example, the lining of the optics of modern weapon platforms, tanks included, is crucial for their performance and may be corroded. Also, in modern tanks, the paint is high-tech and endows the vehicle with both adaptive camouflage and stealth qualities in wide bandwidth, while some antennae for the communication and surveillance systems are embedded in the outer surfaces (Figure 10.1).

Away from the germ and biochemical warfare branches of biowarfare lies the usually neglected realm of macrobiological warfare or bioattack (Kambouris 2021c). This breed bypasses legislation and conventions based on germs and toxins as defining qualities of biowarfare, to the point that foul intention may be suspected from the authors and signatories of such texts and conventions.

The use of animals as agents of warfare can be classified as direct and indirect, as in many other cases, and is ancient. Using a living organism to support one's operations (indirect use) or to directly degrade the enemy capability by disabling personnel, degrading every kind of materiel and disrupting services/procedures (direct use), is attested in many cases through the ages.

In a slightly different context, support functions include numerous examples and applications:

- The use of draught animals to move troops and equipment (Harvey 2018);
- messenger animals, mostly messenger pigeons and dogs (Unknown 2022), to communicate more discreetly than with couriers and messengers;
- guard animals such as guard geese (Boehmer 1986) and guard and patrol dogs (Brice O'Donnell 2014) to secure key locations;
- passive surveillance animals, like canaries and chickens, to detect possibly toxic gases and fumes (Robinson 2003);
- search-and-rescue applications of dogs in the battlefields of WWI (Burton 2020) and in the alpine expansions, with the St. Bernard rescue breed (Blumberg 2016).

Additional uses include the production of biomaterials directly usable for respective purposes—from serpent and insect venom and plant poisons for

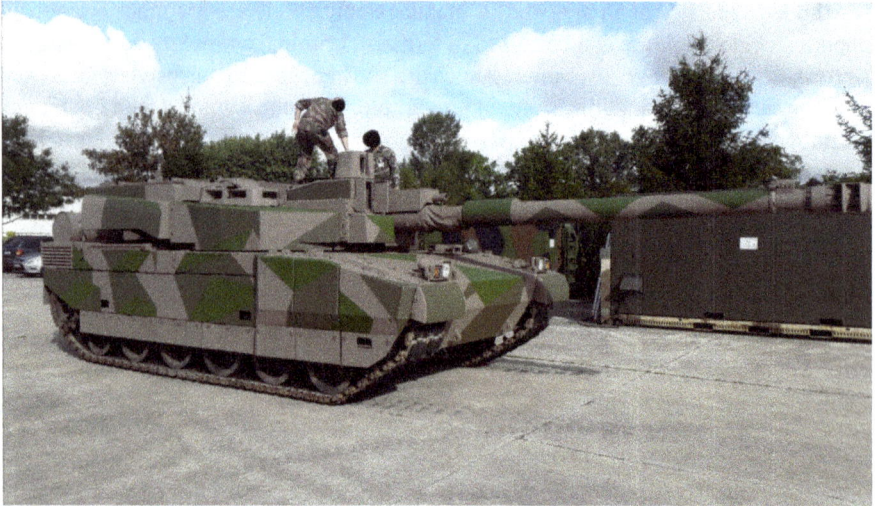

Figure 10.1. The lining in the optics of modern tanks like this French AMX-54 Leclerc is crucial for their performance, while the paint is high-tech and endows the vehicle with (possibly adaptive) camouflage (in the visible and the IR regions of the electromagnetic spectrum) and occasionally with a degree of stealth in radar wavelengths. Furthermore, some antennae for the communications and the surveillance systems are (likely to be) embedded in the outer surfaces. Thus, corrosive bacteria or fungi may degrade both their performance and survivability. (Photo: Nexter®)

assassinations (Pitschmann and Hon 2016) to spider silk for personal protective equipment or body armor (Woody 2020).

Direct employment includes offensive and defensive combat roles. The most basic is the training and use of standard assault wardogs in the past (Brice O'Donnell 2014, Burton 2020); the much more recent examples include bomb-carrying dogs, as used by the Soviets in WWII, to destroy tanks (Aneculaesei 2020), shock cavalry mounts (especially horse and elephants) in many a different military establishment (Kambouris 2023), but especially in Indian, Achaemenid, Hellenistic and Roman ones. Then follows the advent of trained sea animals for detection and guard duty, including intruder neutralization, and for reconnaissance duty in littorals, sea passages and challenging seabed environments, especially to detect mines and different kinds of devices (Unknown n.d. a, Treisman 2022). The use of falconry, previously to intercept messenger animals (MacDonald 2006) and nowadays against small surveillance drones or for suppressing flocks of birds from getting airborne around airbases and causing accidents (MacDonald 2006, Nikolić 2017), is rather less known. Directing clouds of locusts to destroy crops and flights of birds to destroy hot air balloons as well as jets taking off or approaching from very low altitudes (MacDonald 2006) are applications that may or might gain traction in some time.

The common mechanisms and peculiarities in implementation

The different perpetrated bioattack constituents, the 3B, share a common basic mechanism of materialization, but each differs wildly in terms of specifics. There is an overlap and common room in general, but each of the three differ in the mechanistic aspect of threat development and deployment.

The basic, common blueprint is (a) the agent, (b) a delivery means, (c) a vector, and (d) the target. The *agent* is self-explanatory, the *target* less so, despite appearances; the *target* is the entity that is to undergo detrimental (at least in most cases) changes due to the biological function of the agent. It is *not necessarily* (e) the intended effect, as the latter may result indirectly, for instance in the case of severe/unpopular measures imposed to prohibit such detrimental events. An example of the *objective* (intended effect) is the economical mayhem and social upheaval caused by pausing transportation and economic activity in order to contain the spread of a highly infectious, transmittable agent (like SARS-CoV-2) which infects and incapacitates humans (the target).

The *vector* is the entity or procedure that brings the agent to the target in a functional manner under normal, natural conditions. It is the way a bioevent occurs spontaneously, if not intentionally. Vectors are material or procedural entities. The former are generally considered as *carriers*—animate or inanimate. In the case of animate carriers, it is irrespective whether they become affected or remain unaffected by the agent. The notion of inanimate carriers or *fomites* can be expanded to include air, droplets, environmental liquids and solid surfaces.

With regard to vectoring procedures, some references include simple contact (e.g., dermatophytic fungi and various toxins absorbed by the skin like the standard nerve agents/organophosphates), sexual contact (e.g., HIV), inheritance (as occurs with proviruses), injection (e.g., mosquitos transmitting species of the genus *Plasmodium* that cause malaria), inhalation (e.g., SARS-CoV-2), and engulfment/incorporation (e.g., ingress of various toxins through the digestive tract).

The delivery means are exclusive to perpetrated events and refer to the means and processes that bring the agent to the vector in a specific spatio-temporal occurrence and are focal for the success of such endeavors (Nixdorff 2010). Actually, in a more integrated cognitive aspect, the delivery means might be collapsed as a separate stage and be integrated within the vector; in this way, perpetrated and spontaneous events share the same blueprint. In truth, this stage becomes quintessential and defining in the case of perpetrated accidents; the way the accident is engineered actually *is* the delivery means and the accidental process enacts the vectoring phase, although the actual vector remains as discussed above.

In the case of plain, perpetrated events, not disguised as accidents, the most elaborate delivery means can be identified naturally in the realm of biowarfare. They also include the sum of such provisions of biocrime and bioterrorism, due to the nature of warfare as expanded by the introduction of hybrid warfare, which incorporates, among other things, criminal and terrorist applications, virtually unmodified.

Of course, modified military hardware are the warfare-specific delivery amenities; these are mainly shells, missiles and bombs, mostly intended to produce aerosols and possibly other airborne dispersions, as the air ensures the widest distribution to both open and closed spaces, in three-dimensional models, while also allowing transportation to almost all of the points of entry (respiratory tract and the main cover tissue, such as the skin) in both animal and plant species, with few exceptions.

Additionally, contamination of objects and surfaces, and possibly liquid masses (like different bodies of water), allows secondary transmission and the manifestation of secondary infection mechanisms, including access to the digestive tract (by swallowing infected objects or liquids) or through puncture wounds by contaminated sharp, pointed or edged objects (e.g., pebbles, thorns, broken branches, nails or pieces of metal) in urban, suburban or rural environment.

In this respect, the combination of conventional fragmentation weapons with a mechanism of spiking them with a bioagent is expected; it is reminiscent of the empoisoned Scythian arrows from ages past and directly applicable to assassinations, as with the Bulgarian Umbrella, a ricin-injecting mechanism used in London in 1978 (Kambouris and Skiniotis 2021). However, the latter was a targeted, individual assassination weapon rather applicable in crime and terrorism formats and related to warfare only due to the gray, blurred space amongst the 3Bs. The spiking of fragments of bombs, shells and grenades—especially fragmentation models, very common throughout the globe since late 19th century—is yet to occur. Actually, there might be an exception: heat-resistant toxins simply applied (painted) on fragmentation weapons, as occasionally reported for hand grenades issued by the British secret services for the assassination of Reinhard Heydrich in Prague in 1942 (Carus 2002).

However, another approach is the employment of direct dispersion or spraying equipment; it may refer to civil use examples, commandeered or otherwise acquired, or to standard military-grade models. This approach is more efficient, but fraught with considerable drawbacks, such as the easy detection of the carrier and the close range/limited footprint of delivery. Such devices, both military and civil models, may be fixed or mobile, on vehicles of every kind and thus adaptable to terrain, and occasionally airborne as well. Seaborne applications are also possible and, in fact, much easier due to the volume and weight tolerances of vessels compared to airborne and land vehicles (severely limited by gravity and gradients—terrain, contour and altitude, respectively). Such hardware, originally designed for delivery of chemical warfare agents, smoke generation for screening or for firefighting, and occasionally also for crop dusters (the latter, *sensu lato*, is a biosecurity mission), may also be used (Nixdorff 2010).

In warfare, close-range delivery (inherent to biocrime and bioterrorism, applicable by dissolution, local application, injection, etc.) is, as mentioned previously, applicable in the context of hybrid as well as special warfare. Incubation time, meaning the time the weaponized agent needs to start producing results on-target after its delivery there, is critical in this context. However, this parameter is complicated, for there is no consensus in whether the infection process or the appearance of debilitating symptoms (*sensu lato*) is considered as the actual result. In any case, the obvious idea is that from close range use, perhaps from troops-in-contact, immediate results are to be pursued, which rather suggests biochemical warfare, with agents resilient to temperature and thus amenable to application to heated delivery means that can be rudimentarily spiked, such as bullets and fragments of explosive warheads. Massive casualties-causing, long incubation and highly transmittable agents (the SARS-CoV-2 being a prime example, without being necessarily considered a manufactured bioweapon or even used as such) are more applicable to long-distance, strategic-grade warfare.

Such endeavors demand well-timed use of local delivery agents (such as friendly agents pre-existing in sufficient numbers), appropriate disposition and suitable distribution on the enemy ground or enjoying freedom of movement. Thus, to allow them the conclusion of a massive, planned dispersion/delivery attempt and possibly time to egress themselves from the danger zone, a delay in infection and onset of symptoms is quintessential. This approach is stealthy, allows deniability and renders irrelevant the elaborate defense systems such as the currently developed beam (generally laser) weapons (Figure 10.2) intended to destroy high-speed, small and medium size incoming projectiles possibly containing Weapons of Mass Destruction (WMD) for local, stand-in release.

The other, much more conventional mechanism is by long-range (stealth or otherwise) delivery systems carried on projectiles, such as hyperguns, long-range ballistic missiles with or without gliding terminal effectors, long-range aircraft or drones/UAVs, cruise missiles and, last but not least, orbital bombing systems. Some of the above are inherently, or may be, used clandestinely—or at least with some stealth. In the former case, it is to deny resilience and reaction, as well as accountability and retaliation, whereas in the latter case, it is only to degrade resilience so as to shrink the window of countermeasures (Kambouris and Georgoulas 2021, Kambouris et al. 2021), especially since new technologies, including beam weapons (Figure 10.2), seem to gain advantage and be prone to achieving credible interception.

However, the reverse arrangement is also conceivable and makes perfect sense. By employing delayed-action agents, troops in contact may clear the infected area, thus exposing the advancing enemy elements, if this application is followed in retreat—genuine or fake. In case of advance, the use of delayed-action bioweapons, coupled with issuing antidotes and other countermeasures to own troops and assets (including antibiotics), allows the purging of the occupied ground infested by the

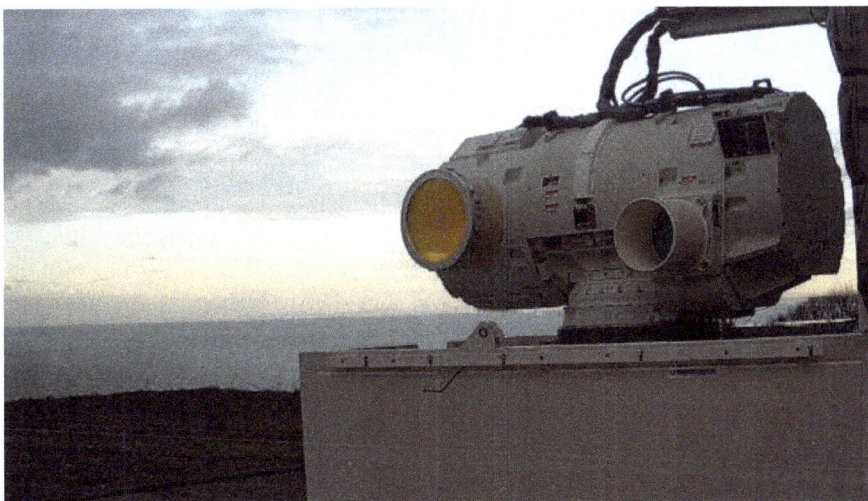

Figure 10.2. Laser beam weapon "Dragonfire" intended for the prompt and repeated destruction of small flying or gliding threats, from mini drones to missiles and projectiles, so as to nullify saturation and reduce the involuntary dispersal of any possible agent caused by the usual 'dynamic neutralization' of the carrier (i.e., by blowing it up). (Photo: MBDA®)

remaining or hiding enemy elements, such as guerillas and special operators. On the other hand, prompt action agents delivered massively, at a great distance, may crush the enemy morale and severely undermine the resistance potential of a prospective foe or declared enemy.

Biocrime and bioterrorism events may use elaborate or crude techniques to deliver agents, from widely available dispersion/spraying equipment (for example, models used in gardening) to commercially available and crudely modified UAV/UGV to hand applications by paint brush and syringes.

The 5G networks, pertaining to all surveillance equipment and all personal devices, allow to the controllers of such networks a -controversial- means to survey 60/24/7 against, and timely respond to, such events. Or at least they provide a window and an object for reaction even retrospectively, so as to ensure accountability and thus ascertain future deterrence. In this respect, the nature of respective agents and operatives becomes of the utmost importance. In both cases, enemy state special operators and local criminally-disposed elements are a natural human resource. But, especially in acts of terrorism, recruitment may occur massively amongst dissident/disenfranchised natives and, more easily and readily so, among indoctrinated resident aliens (the latter taken to imply differences in any or both of pedigree/origin and culture/values) approached either beforehand, at their loci of origin, or on the spot, after being set or even settled at their destinations, intentional or circumstantial.

In terms of mechanistic planning and implementation, drone technology (actually UAVs), especially coupled with Artificial Intelligence (AI), change(s) the map (Figure 10.3). Still, as a rule, *crime* suggests small-scale targeted delivery from close range, whereas *warfare* implies a rather long-range and massive dispersal over extended areas. *Terrorism* may use both these approaches, depending mainly on the kind of terrorism and its target. Eliminating individual, high-prestige targets such as dignitaries, heads of state and high-status celebrities or scientific and corporate personalities, or key agents, such as the prominent members of an operational (military or otherwise) chain-of-command, verges on crime. On the other hand, attempting to orchestrate mass events is more akin to warfare, with the notable exception that, in terms of execution, such attempts tend to be implemented in close proximity.

Mass migration and the volume of trade (at least pre-COVID-19) tend to nullify a very clear distinction; where terrorism was *mainly* performed within the borders of a state, a crime was *definitely* within the borders and warfare *always* spreads across the, or some kind of, borders, impacting at least two parties/states directly. The idea of borders could be functional rather than legal, in order to signify the controlled or directly occupied territory, and should be understood as a more or less linear separation. The legal status of warfare, which implies declaration of war, may not be applicable here, and the concept was expanded to include non-state actors, especially based in failed states, as a definite footprint is necessary to conceptualize the separation and thus transgression. Now, borders may not separate conflicting populations which may well occupy intermingled ground footprint, as, in many cases, mass migration has been occurring, despite the lack of amicable relations (or even in the presence of extreme friction and prejudice bordering outright enmity) between the migrating and the host populations. An open conflict would be simply an asymmetrical, hybrid warfare—the latter especially so if it devolves to the use

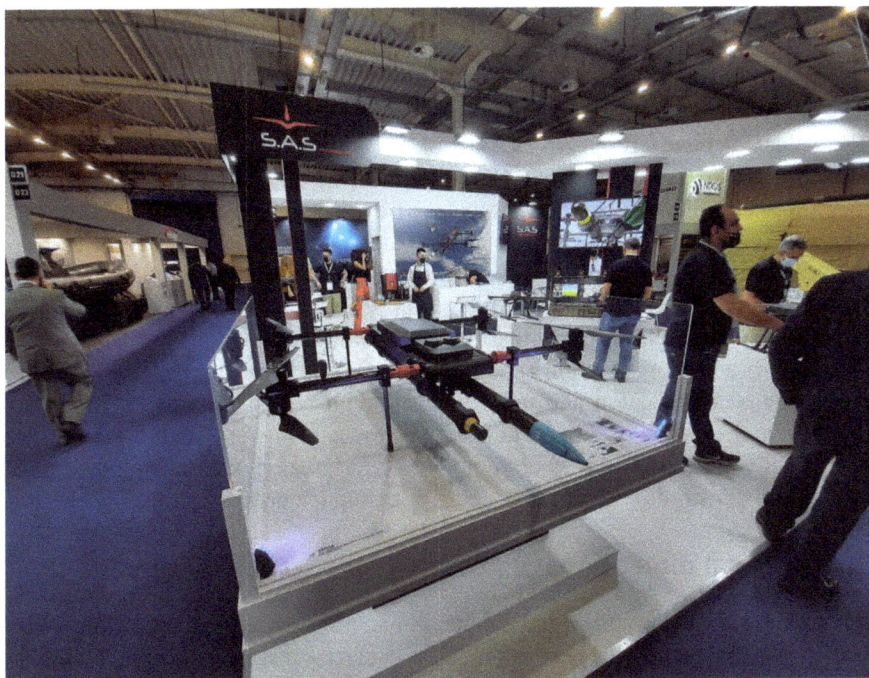

Figure 10.3. Weaponized UAVs of relatively small size may deliver, with the accuracy of conventional weapons (in this case, the standard 2.75" unguided Hydra-70 rockets), small but lethal loads of dispersible bioagents, thus featuring scalable destructivity, depending on the exact nature of the target and the agent used. (Photo: D. Stergiou, with permission)

of bioagents—without the spatial distinction and discrimination that allow the development of resilience, especially surveillance.

A state-sponsored, massive event (massive in terms of scale of impact and/or perpetration) is an act of war, with functional characteristics indiscernible from an act of terrorism. This is especially so if the scale is kept relatively small, preferably by limiting the number of agents/perpetrators involved. This approach is indeed facilitated by the universal availability and accessibility of small, commercial drones and their modification for rather sinister uses.

Long-range exchange of biological strikes is conceivable, but the greater number of actual conflicts is prone to be local; in hybrid warfare formats long-range endeavors are likely to be assigned to state or non-state proxies. As the scales are of no particular help, and nor is geography, whether a given event is crime, terrorism or warfare may be controversial and resolvable only by the identification of the beneficiary of the occurrence of the perpetrated event. The cooperation of more than one such parties, of different legal status, may complicate things even further. Profound deliberation is needed to decide the optimal solution in the matter: One approach is to assign a mixed, multiple designation to a given event, to correspond with all the perpetrators. Another approach is to develop a mechanism of reduction to a common denominator for all involved parties.

Then, there is the spontaneous/accidental dimension. Although directly opposite to the perpetrated one, in sense and practicality, there is an interesting overlap. It refers to the intentional actions or to the intentional failure to do so, intended to cause accidents resulting in the release of bioagents or an increase in their adverse impact. The failure of biosafety measures, possibly in Wuhan 2019 (Holmes et al. 2021) and definitely in Sverdlovsk 1979 (Kambouris 2018), is the commonest ground for such instances, although the advancement of bioeconomy (Aguilar et al. 2019) is expected to multiply the levels, instances and occurrences of such events. Errors occurring intentionally in synthetic biology or more basic biotechnological risks may cause extinction level events more easily than before due to the sheer scale of near-future bioprocesses, from biomining (Cockell et al. 2020), bioaugmentation (Nzila et al. 2016) and biorestoration (Satijn and de Boks 1988) to terraforming, waste processing/recapitalization and mass production/processing of edibles. This does not include the spread of disease to people and assets of every kind; the disruption of productive processes, based on biology to a far greater extent than today, when synthetic chemistry is still supreme, could be disruptive on a disastrous scale.

The practical dimensions of preparedness against biothreats

The recent events from Libya to Ukraine, through Syria and Yemen, just prove that wars—in all but name—are here to stay: "the sad fact is that international politics has always been a ruthless and dangerous business, and it is likely to remain that way" (Mearsheimer 2001).

Concerning the future, the classification of tomorrow's conflicts in terms applied on the basis of historical lessons learned seems inadequate as a scientific approach. The evolving nature of conflict, which is best characterized by convergence, makes doubtful the applicability of clear-cut distinctions that were needed to plan accordingly using just as clear-cut algorithms and SOPs. Irrespective of the term used—'compound', 'hybrid', 'unconventional', 'irregular', '2nd generation' or '3rd generation', which may be applicable for the theory of conflict, the grim reality will still be that any and all of the aforementioned conflict types, potentially and probably combined with crime and terrorism (Kondylis 2007), will produce a very complex future reality. A reality that must favor stability rather than total prevalence against an enemy (individual humans or groups such as non-state actors, state agents, state-sponsored groups, etc.), similarly to Cold War ethics. While the concrete knowledge of Mutually Assured Destruction (MAD) made stability the only option in the past, the same deadlock approaches today for very different reasons. It is the actual *deficit of knowledge* that promotes stability over prevalence, since deterring or preventing or prevailing against the unknown is absurd as a notion, especially when taking into consideration biological threats.

Deterrence is considered as the primary defensive tool of small countries against powerful ones, but it also provides a determined balance in order to avoid conflict amongst highly powerful forces (Seidman and Alexander 2008). It roots from the opponent's fear of unbearable costs from the possible escalation of conflict between the two sides. The biological agents, although in theory the quintessence of the

Weapon of Mass Distraction (WMD) category, cannot serve as a valid deterrent in practice. They bioweapons are unstable, especially germs (communicable germs), for they can be contained only with extreme difficulty from the moment one single individual is infected and becomes itself infective (infection zero). Repercussions ranging from the global public opinion and extending, through legal prohibitions, up to climactic response by other WMD, combine with the very questionable reliability of bioweapons, to dissuade their use, especially in the smaller countries' deterrence plans.

The other possible option—prevention—is a very promising one according to official documents and literature among policymakers and think tanks. In essence, prevention has a weak case concerning biothreats for three simple reasons. The first reason, owing to the fog of the future, is the inability to accurately foretell, while even small divergence and inaccuracy in forecast may bear extreme results. The paradigm is that one plane (arguably massive, Boeing B-29 bomber) slipping through was all the difference in the nuclear bombing of Hiroshima (Unknown n.d b). Additionally, the temperamental engine of an Aichi E13A recon seaplane caused the defeat of the Japanese in Midway (Cox 2019).

The second reason stems from the fact that the friction of engagement may turn chaotic, as goes the motto of Von Moltke the Elder (Moltke and Hughes 2009). The third reason is that every effort meant to preemptively tackle an enemy threat is inherently limited, due to the design principles of basic military offensive operations and thus contestable by enemy counter-planning. Accordingly, preparedness turns out to be the only feasible option in our efforts to face any potential biological threat.

In the struggle against pandemics—spontaneous or perpetrated —societies will always be better prepared tomorrow than today, but never enough. All the critical infrastructure (like laboratories, hospitals, communication facilities and procedures) among the involved agencies and their personnel are a priority as are the military, security and response infrastructure and personnel, that consist strategic assets of low availability and high demand, difficult to replace and not expendable.

Of course, the armed forces—the key player in large-scale conflicts, by definition—are of paramount importance; still, they must cooperate with other agencies in order to pool resources to achieve adequacy of means. Subsequently, it would be possible to organize a multi-agency network to run and support operations for the protection and recovery of the threatened entities, military and civilian alike. However, such an interaction may cause friction and, owing to the inability to properly communicate, which is a very complicated and risky proposition during a crisis, actually become counter-productive. Nevertheless, the COVID-19 pandemic suggests that in a biological crisis, the centralized, total-resource approach can be successful, as shown by the early example of China in Wuhan. The government-ordained local center of operations, with specialized scientists, officers and technocrats pooling holistic knowledge of the causes, events, means and their capabilities, might outperform the nimble and lean-and-mean military Joint Operations Center (JOC) concepts of American-trained and indoctrinated organizations.

Containment, tracking/surveillance and enforcement measures raise issues of compliance with the existing legal framework for human rights. There are, however, certain provisions not only in the UN Human Rights Charter but also in the recently enacted GDPR of the European Union (EU 2016), which legitimize security protocols when it comes to the handling of health crisis situations.

In the military world and way of thinking, the assets better poised to counter a given threat within a projected operational environment (OE) are the prime targets, as their degradation or elimination would allow a free reign to any perpetrator using any given means of assault and thus maximize the destructive potential of any combination. The capabilities and vulnerabilities of such assets are a primary concern that the enemy or the perpetrator takes into account in their planning process. The Comprehensive Preparation of the Operational Environment (CPOE), that is, the analytical procedure with intelligence input undertaken by a staff to support the decision-making process (Unknown 2019), needs, above all, to secure the responders, whose survivability, readiness, resilience and mobility are considered vital.

Bibliography

Aguilar, A. et al. (2019). Bioeconomy for sustainable development. Biotechnology Journal. Biotechnol J, 14(8). doi: 10.1002/BIOT.201800638.

Aneculaesei, C. (2020). The Soviet Anti-Tank Dog. How the Soviets used man's best friend, History of Yesterday. Available at: https://historyofyesterday.com/the-soviet-anti-tank-dog-7f00425652eb (Accessed: 5 August 2022).

Belandis, D. (2004). Humanitary intervention and terrorism. *In*: Takis, A.C. and Manitakis, A.N. (eds.). Terrosism and Rights. Athens: Savvalas Publications.

Blumberg, J. (2016). A Brief History of the St. Bernard Rescue Dog, Travel, Smithsonian Magazine. Available at: https://www.smithsonianmag.com/travel/a-brief-history-of-the-st-bernard-rescue-dog-13787665/ (Accessed: 5 August 2022).

Boehmer, G. (1986). US Military Installations Using Goose Guards | AP News, Acissiated Press. Available at: https://apnews.com/article/4d88d888221a417cefffcff7743a5789 (Accessed: 5 August 2022).

Boltsis, I. et al. (2021). The genomic dimension in Biodefense: Decontamination. pp. 197–218. *In*: Kambouris, M. (ed.). Genomics in Biosecurity. 1st edn. London: ELSEVIER ACADEMIC PRESS.

Brice O'Donnell, K. (2014). Military working dogs, past, present and future | History and Policy, History and Policy. Available at: https://www.historyandpolicy.org/opinion-articles/articles/military-working-dogs-past-present-and-future (Accessed: 5 August 2022).

Britannica. (no date a). Assassins. Available at: https://www.britannica.com/story/who-were-the-assassins (Accessed: 10 August 2022).

Britannica. (no date b). Templar. Available at: https://www.britannica.com/topic/Templars (Accessed: 10 August 2022)

Britannica. (no date c). East India Company. Available at: https://www.britannica.com/topic/East-India-Company (Accessed: 10 August 2022).

Britannica. (no date d). Dutch West India Company. Available at: https://www.britannica.com/topic/Dutch-West-India-Company (Accessed: 10 August 2022).

Burton, J. (2020). The Casualty Dogs of World War I, The History Reader. Available at: https://www.thehistoryreader.com/historical-fiction/the-casualty-dogs-of-world-war-i/ (Accessed: 5 August 2022).

Carus, W.S. (2002). Bioterrorism and Biocrimes: The Illicit Use of Biological Agents Since 1900. Amsterdam: Fredonia Books.

Cockell, C.S. et al. (2020). Space station biomining experiment demonstrates rare earth element extraction in microgravity and Mars gravity. Nature Communications, 11(1): 1–11. doi: 10.1038/s41467-020-19276-w.

Cox, S.J. (2019). 'ISR' (Intelligence, Surveillance and Reconnaissance) in the Battle of Midway, Navy League. Available at: https://www.navyleaguewestct.org/ISR at the Battle of Midway.pdf (Accessed: 12 August 2022).

Dawson, W. (1925). The Mouse in Fable and Folklore on JSTOR. Folclore, 36(3): 227–248.

European Union 2016 Regulation (EU) 2016/679 of The European Parliament and of The Council of April 27, 2016. Available at: https://www.eumonitor.eu/9353000/1/j4nvk6yhcbpeywk_j9vvik7m1c3gyxp/vk3t7p3lbczq (Accessed: 16 January 2023).

Ganor, B. (2010). Defining terrorism: Is One Man's Terrorist another Man's Freedom Fighter? Police Practice and Research, 3(4): 287–304. doi: 10.1080/1561426022000032060.

Gottschalk, R. and Preiser, W. (2005). Bioterrorism: Is it a real threat? Med Microbiol Immunol, 194(3): 109–14. doi: 10.1007/s00430-004-0228-z.

Harvey, I. (2018). Unusual Warriors - Animal Roles in the Military, War History Online. Available at: https://www.warhistoryonline.com/war-articles/animals-in-war.html?edg-c=1 (Accessed: 5 August 2022).

Hoffman, B. (2017). Inside terrorism. Columbia University Press.

Holmes, E.C. et al. (2021). The origins of SARS-CoV-2: A critical review. Cell, 184(19): 4848–4856. doi: 10.1016/J.CELL.2021.08.017.

Kambouris, M.E. (2021a). Global catastrophic biological risks: Nature and response. pp. 29–42. *In:* Kambouris, M.E. (ed.). Genomics in Biosecurity. 1st edn. London: Elsevier Academic Press.

Kambouris, M.E. (2021b). The concept of humanome and the microbiomic dimension. pp. 15–28. *In:* Kambouris, M. (ed.). Genomics in Biosecurity. 1st edn. London: Elsevier Academic Press.

Kambouris, M.E. (2021c). Exploring the concepts: Biosecurity, biodefence and biovigilance. pp. 3–14. *In:* Kambouris, M.E. (ed.). Genomics in Biosecurity. 1st edn. London: Elsevier Academic Press.

Kambouris, M.E. (2023). Alexander the great Avenger. Barnsley: Pen & Sword Military.

Kambouris, M.E. (2018). Mobile stand-off and stand-in surveillance against biowarfare and bioterrorism agents. pp. 241–55. *In:* Karampelas, P. and Bourlai, T. (eds.). Advanced Sciences and Technologies for Security Applications. Springer. doi: 10.1007/978-3-319-68533-5_12.

Kambouris, M.E. et al. (2018). Rebooting bioresilience: A Multi-OMICS approach to tackle global catastrophic biological risks and next-generation biothreats. OMICS A Journal of Integrative Biology, 22(1): 35–51. doi: 10.1089/omi.2017.0185.

Kambouris, M.E. et al. (2021). Biodefense build 2.0: The muscle. pp. 167–182. *In:* Kambouris, M.E. (ed.). Genomics in Biosecurity. 1st edn. London: Elsevier Academic Press.

Kambouris, M.E. and Georgoulas, D. (2021). Bio-offense: Technical means, tactical approaches, operational orientations, and strategic concepts. pp. 127–142. *In:* Kambouris, M.E. (ed.). Genomics in Biosecurity. 1st edn. London: Elsevier Academic Press.

Kambouris, M.E. and Skiniotis, G. (2021). Nonmicrobial biothreats: DNA, prions, and (bio)regulators/(bio) toxins. pp. 75–91. *In:* Kambouris, M. (ed.). Genomics in Biosecurity. 1st edn. London: ELSEVIER ACADEMIC PRESS.

Kip, N. and Van Veen, J.A. (2015). The dual role of microbes in corrosion. The ISME Journal, 9(3): 542. doi: 10.1038/ISMEJ.2014.169.

Kondylis, P. (2007). The political and the Man. Athens: Themelio.

Lechner, S. (2017). Anarchy in International Relations, Oxford Research Encyclopedia of International Studies. Oxford University Press. doi: 10.1093/ACREFORE/9780190846626.013.79.

MacDonald, H. (2006). Falcon. Reaktion B. London.

Mearsheimer, J.J. (2001). The tragedy of great power politics. NEW YORK: W. W. Norton & Co.

Moltke, H. and Hughes, D.J. (2009). Moltke on the art of war : Selected writings. Random House Publishing Group.

Nikolić, S.S. (2017). An innovative response to commercial UAV menace-anti-UAV falconry. Vojno Delo, 4: 146–167. doi: 10.5937/vojdelo1704146N.

Nixdorff, K. (2010). Advances in targeted delivery and the future of bioweapons: Bulletin of the Atomic Scientists, 66(1): 24–33. doi: 10.2968/066001004.

Nzila, A. et al. (2016). Bioaugmentation: An emerging strategy of industrial wastewater treatment for reuse and discharge. International Journal of Environmental Research and Public Health, 13(9). doi: 10.3390/IJERPH13090846.

Pitschmann, V. and Hon, Z. (2016). Military importance of natural toxins and their analogs. Molecules, 21: 556. doi: 10.3390/molecules21050556.

Robinson, S. (2003). Chickens to be used by u.s. military to detect deadly chemicals in Iraq, United Poultry Concerns. Available at: https://www.upc-online.org/alerts/021903ChickenDefense.htm (Accessed: 5 August 2022).

Satijn, H.M.C. and de Boks, P.A. (1988). Biorestoration, a Technique for Remedial Action on Industrial Sites. Contaminated Soil '88. Springer, Dordrecht, pp. 745–753. doi: 10.1007/978-94-009-2807-7_120.

Seidman, S. and Alexander, J.C. (eds.). (2008). The New Social Theory Reader: Contemporary debates. 2nd edn. London: Routledge. doi: 10.4324/9781003060963/NEW-SOCIAL-THEORY-READER-STEVEN-SEIDMAN-JEFFREY-ALEXANDER.

Sowmyya, T. (2011). Crime: A conceptual understanding. Indian Journal of Applied Research, 4(3): 196–198. doi: 10.15373/2249555X/MAR2014/58.

Treisman, R. (2022). A Russian naval base is defended by dolphins. It's not as unusual as it sounds, National Public Radio. Available at: https://text.npr.org/1095549251 (Accessed: 10 August 2022).

Unknown. (2019). Allied Joint Doctrine for the Planning of Operations Edition A Version 2, UK Change 1. (Accessed: 10 August 2022).

Unknown. (2022). The Incredible Carrier Pigeons of the First World War Imperial War Museums. Available at: https://www.iwm.org.uk/history/the-incredible-carrier-pigeons-of-the-first-world-war (Accessed: 5 August 2022).

Unknown. (no date a). A Combat Divers Worst Nightmare Navy SEALs. Available at: https://navyseals.com/2210/a-combat-divers-worst-nightmare-marine-mammal-program/(Accessed: 5   August 2022).

Unknown. (no date b). The Atomic Bombings of Hiroshima and Nagasaki. Available at: https://www.atomicarchive.com/resources/documents/med/med_chp7.html (Accessed: 16 January 2023).

Wikipedia. (no date). Banana Republic. Available at: https://en.wikipedia.org/wiki/Banana_republic (Accessed: 16 January 2023).

Woody, C. (2020) High-tech body armor of the future could come from spider butts, We Are The Mighty. Available at: https://www.wearethemighty.com/mighty-trending/body-armor-spider-silk/ (Accessed: 10 August 2022).

Index

A

Agrosecurity 16–21, 24, 25
agroterrorism 16–20
archaeological chemistry 6
Artificial Intelligence-AI 120, 129
Astrobiology 51–54, 57

B

Bacteriophages 112, 113
Big Data 121
biochemical warfare 154, 155, 158
biocrime 154, 157, 158, 160
biocybernetics 114, 115
bioeconomy 16, 22, 23, 119, 124
biologicals 107, 111, 112
biomolecular archaeology 6, 12
biopharmaceuticals 108, 110–112
bioregulators 109, 111
Biosociomics 1, 13
bioterrorism 154, 157, 158, 160
biotoxins 111, 113, 115
biowarfare/biological warfare 153–155, 157
blockchain 30

C

COVID-19 38–41
cyberbiosecurity 119, 120, 122–124, 126–130

E

eDNA 67
electroculturomics 139–141
electrogenomics 140
electromagnetic amenities 133, 144
electromicrobiology 135, 136, 141
electronic health record 127
electrostimulation 133–135, 137, 140
Electrotranscriptomics 140
emerging foodborne pathogens 31
emerging pathogens 70, 71, 77

evolutionary emergence 71, 74, 81
Exobiology 51–55, 57
exogenome 67, 77, 79

F

food authentication 34, 38
food fraud 31, 34–38
food safety 29–41
functional emergence 71, 76, 80

G

genetic pollution 20
Geobiology 52, 53
germ warfare 154
germ-ganism 94, 95, 99–101, 103, 104, 109–111, 113, 116, 134, 137, 141–143

H

host species barrier 24

I

Iatromics 5, 12, 13
Information Technologies-IT 122, 127
intensive farming 17, 25
Internet of Things-IoT 121

L

Lateral Gene Transfer 75, 77
long range transcellular communication 93

M

microbiome 110–112, 116

N

non-contact cell-to-cell interaction 93

O

Ohmic effects 136

P

paleogenomics 6, 7, 11, 12
paleomicrobiology 6–8, 10, 12
paleopathology 5–8, 12
physical emergence 71
prevention 163

R

risk assessment 30, 35–37

S

Shadow Biosphere 50–52, 54, 58
synthetic biology 120, 123, 125

T

tumor-ganism 101

V

virophages 112, 113

X

Xenobiology 50–55, 57, 58, 60–62
Xenobiota compatibility score 57

For Product Safety Concerns and Information please contact our EU
representative GPSR@taylorandfrancis.com
Taylor & Francis Verlag GmbH, Kaufingerstraße 24, 80331 München, Germany